LABOURS
OF LOVE

Also by Madeleine Bunting

NON-FICTION

Love of Country: A Hebridean Journey

The Plot: A Biography of an English Acre

Willing Slaves: How the Overwork
Culture is Ruling Our Lives

The Model Occupation: The Channel
Islands under German Rule 1940–45

FICTION

Island Song

LABOURS OF LOVE

The Crisis of Care

MADELEINE BUNTING

GRANTA

Granta Publications, 12 Addison Avenue, London W11 4QR
First published in Great Britain by Granta Books, 2020

A CIP catalogue record for this book
is available from the British Library.

1 3 5 7 9 10 8 6 4 2

ISBN 978 1 78378 379 3
eISBN 978 1 78378 380 9

Typeset in Caslon by M Rules
Printed and bound by CPI Group (UK) Ltd, Croydon, CR0 4YY

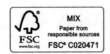

MIX
Paper from
responsible sources
FSC® C020471
www.fsc.org

Contents

Author's Note

The proofs for this book arrived at the same time as the global Covid-19 crisis erupted. London had fallen deathly silent except for the wail of sirens. Our household, like many others, was in quarantine after my daughter had fallen sick. In ways beyond my wildest imaginings, the themes of this book had been thrust to the forefront of everyone's minds.

Suddenly and dramatically, in the shadow of this global pandemic, we have all become acutely aware of our physical vulnerability, our dependence on others for care, our appreciation of those whose job it is to care, and our own role in caring. Over the last five years of research, I had been investigating a 'quiet crisis buried in individual lives' (p. 5), but in March 2020 we faced the opposite: a crisis of care which has brought our daily lives and the world economy to a juddering, disorientating halt. Covid-19 has starkly exposed the chronic underinvestment and undervaluing of care; in the relatively early days of this crisis, the outlook is that the UK's precarious and overstretched health and social care systems will buckle, and as a result, thousands of lives will be lost. As the pandemic progresses and hopefully passes, Covid-19 will unleash a huge questioning of the politics and governing systems which failed to foresee this disaster. That could lead to anger, but equally, could trigger a massive cultural shift in which we come to recognize the foundations of care on which all human wellbeing rests. How we organize and fund health and social care could be transformed. We have been brutally reminded that the marginalization of people – the homeless, asylum seekers, prisoners in crowded jails– will contribute to the severity of the pandemic. For the first time ever in human history, no one is immune, every human being is in this together. The tragedy is that it has taken a disaster to understand our commonality.

Government announcements during the pandemic have repeatedly used the word 'essential' when referring to our caring services. As we experience multiple restrictions on our daily life, we are learning fast the meaning of that word. Lockdown is an entirely novel experience for many in rich countries whose lives are full of complexity, freedom, opportunity and luxury. Suddenly we realize that what is essential is care, and our greatest nightmares are its absence. Will there be nurses and doctors? Will there be beds and equipment? If I am scared who will hold my hand? For those at home the questions are no less urgent. Who is on hand to bring us food? Who can fetch medications? Networks of care are springing up around us as I write; my phone reverberates with messages from my street WhatsApp group: offers to help with shopping and to share food and medicine. Meanwhile, Covid-19 has revealed a humbling truth: that our measures of status and value are flimsy, and that it is the low-paid labour of cleaners, supermarket assistants, and social care workers that is essential. They will be the ones keeping us fed and safe, thus saving lives.

Through much of this book runs an argument about the invisibility of care, and its historic under-valuing. Covid-19 has upended this: care has suddenly taken centre stage. I hope that my investigation can contribute to the soul searching that will follow this crisis; the cry of 'why did no one see this coming?', as the Queen asked after the 2008 financial crisis. Over the last decade, we have stripped care systems to the bone – not just health and social care – but in neighbourhoods so that people have lost the habit of asking or offering help. What has made those threadbare care systems so dangerous is that at the same time, medical advances have extended lives so that a greater proportion of the population have fragile health. Covid-19 ripped into the gap I describe in chapter one between the growing need for care and the inadequate systems available to provide it.

A wide-ranging global debate will follow this pandemic for years to come, and this book will play its part by defining what we overlooked. It throws light on many of the attributes, activities and people we will need to value afresh. I can see a new politics of care emerging which recognizes our interdependence as families, friends, communities, towns, cities, nations and as a human species. Terrifying though these days are, we are witnessing a dramatic global effort to save lives. That is inspiring. Everywhere people are focused on this one task, whether they are overworked hospital doctors, engineers building ventilators, scientists researching vaccines or the billions who are staying at home. We are being reminded of what matters: both life and what sustains it, care.

Madeleine Bunting
March 2020

Introduction

Each of us has been shaped by the care of others. From the
first touch of the midwife's worn hands as she pulled you into
the world, your life has been sustained by a long catalogue of
people who have nurtured and supported your development
and well-being up to this point. Ahead lie more experiences of
being cared for, possibly from those you love and certainly from
many strangers, whom you may completely depend on for your
most basic needs for comfort, food and cleanliness. No one can
afford not to be interested in care.

We need a better understanding of this small word, of the
motivation to provide care, and of the skills and knowledge
required. Some of this labour takes place within the family:
parents care for their children, siblings for each other, and, to a
varying extent, children for their parents. Some care is threaded
into friendships, romantic love and between neighbours. For
millions of people, care has become a job, which requires

quickly establishing trust and empathy over the course of busy shifts in a care home, doctor's surgery or on a hospital ward.

Care is the critical element of some professions, and at the same time is referred to as a business, even an industry. A few pockets of this work are highly prestigious – brain surgery, for example – while some hold huge significance in our lives, such as the care woven into intimacy. But much is concerned with the daily maintenance of human welfare, which all too easily slips from view and is taken for granted.

Yet chances are that most people find themselves providing care during their life, and for women, in particular, it can become an all-consuming task for months or years. Care relationships involve knotty issues of dependence, vulnerability, intimacy, risk, resentment, and fulfilment. Some people come to this life lesson young – around 180,000 children under eighteen in the UK are carers; for many others, their induction is parenting, but it could be the sickness of a partner or friend, or the ageing of one's own parents – care that can now last decades. Every year, 2.1 million adults in the UK take on the care of an elderly or disabled relative (and approximately the same number find that role comes to an end). The care of the elderly and long-term sick enlists one in eight of the UK adult population (6.5 million), and their numbers are expected to grow by 40 per cent in the next twenty years.

The vast work of care, both unpaid and paid, still predominantly falls to women. All my life – I was born in 1964 – women have been challenging the stereotypes which have defined their lives. They have claimed their right to work outside the home, to pursue careers and to win financial independence, yet care is still seen as women's work. They are still responsible for a larger share of parenting and housework, and a disproportionate number find themselves also caring for parents and for their partners. As lives lengthen, one in four women in their fifties and sixties will take on a care role and their numbers are rising fast. By the age of fifty-nine, women will have a fifty-fifty chance of being, or having been, a carer for a sick or elderly person. At the same time, many are still raising their teenage children and almost half of those over fifty-five are providing regular care for grandchildren. This midway point in life is laden with acute awareness of the growing vulnerabilities of elderly parents, while dealing with the needs of children and young adults. Middle age for women can entail the most intense labour of care of their lives. 'Sandwich carer' is a phrase that inadequately conveys the painful pull to provide care to different generations, perhaps seventy-odd years apart, with a motorway journey of several hours between – as I have discovered from experience while writing this book. After providing all this care, women's longer life expectancy often means they find themselves alone – without the care of a partner – in the final years of their lives.

This gendered pattern of care is also stubbornly evident in the workforce. Women dominate caring professions such as nursing (89 per cent), social work (75 per cent), and childcare (98 per cent). They now form the majority of GPs (54 per cent) and three out of four teachers are female. And they provide the vast bulk of the army of healthcare workers in the NHS (80 per cent) and social-care workers (82 per cent) for the long-term sick, disabled and frail elderly. In recent decades, these percentages have barely shifted, despite the myriad changes in women's lives over that time, and some have become even more marked. The proportion of women in general practice jumped 12 per cent in the decade 2007 to 2017. Men play a crucial role in care – as fathers, husbands, nurses and doctors, amongst many other roles – but that can't obscure the persistence of this gender imbalance. Care is *the* feminist issue; it profoundly shapes women's lives at home and at work.

Despite the scale of the immense labour of care, there is a

cultural blindness to it, a profound refusal to recognize and value the work that sustains human well-being. Making visible the nature of this vast web of care – its importance, extent, subtlety and complexity – is the purpose of this book. Our society does not invest time, money or value in the care economy, nor does it recognize its currency of time, attention, empathy, respect, trust, dignity, reciprocity and solidarity. It does not acknowledge how good care depends on a wider context of decent pay and working conditions, adequate funding, effective organizations and cultural recognition. Despite persistent mythologies to the contrary, care is not the work of saints, angels and heroic individuals.

We have reached a juncture where a collision of long-term historical trends and contemporary politics is provoking a crisis of care. Aspects of the crisis surface in political life – the scandal of inadequate social care or the collapsing mental-health care system – and reports are commissioned, and inquiries produce sensible recommendations. But words pile up without effective action as the crisis is caught in a repetitive loop of alarm alternating with apathy. Frequently, it is women in both their personal and their working lives who are left to cope with the consequences of this crisis, as they stretch their own resources, emotional and physical, to reduce its impact on those they are caring for.

I wish a fraction of the energy and profile of the Me Too movement could find its counterpart exposing this care deficit. The subject struggles for public attention, crippled by a long history of invisibility and complacency. In the UK, budget cuts in the name of austerity have reduced already inadequate services, and more than a generation of chronic underinvestment is only acknowledged (if at all) in the aftermath of a shocking scandal. Risk and dependence underlie all relationships of care, so the subject is instinctively feared, but scandal leads to more regulation and inspection, and rarely to the increased funding needed to reduce workloads and improve training. This under-investment costs lives and brings untold suffering and stress to millions, both to those offering care and to those needing it. A quiet crisis is buried in individual lives, its fallout often characterized as personal failure.

Care has many elements: it may require expert knowledge and skill, it may entail insight, creativity and empathy, but, equally, it may be routine and repetitive. Professor Alison Leary, a mathematician and nurse, argues that care can only be understood in terms of complexity theory, because it involves so many variables and the relationships between them are so complex. 'You can't pigeonhole it – it has multiple meanings, because it is always situational and contextual,' she told me over coffee, laughing at my deepening frown. I had set out to analyse and define the word, and had stumbled into its large empire of meanings. Often the language of care seemed to collapse under the weight of what people were trying to describe to me. Partly, this is because so much of care is grounded in tacit knowledge: it is felt and touched, rather than articulated in words. Partly, it is because the language has become worn and hollowed-out of meaning. At the end of every chapter, I explore a word closely associated care, drawing on its etymology to find a keyhole into the cultural assumptions which have patterned our understanding. In recent decades, care has been swamped by new languages – commercial, consumer or managerial – which threaten the essence of what is at stake: it is referred to as an 'industry', or a 'business sector', yet it is rooted in solidarity and ethics. The low-paid healthcare assistant who turns up on the ward for a twelve-hour shift of feeding, washing and changing beds is the product of centuries of ethical philosophy, politics, economics and religious ideals.

*

I criss-crossed the country from north to south, east to west, to meet people who were caring for others. I sat in meetings and followed people around; I listened and watched. It proved harder to get access than I had imagined. Outside scrutiny is harsh, and organizations were reluctant, and I'm grateful to all those who agreed to take the risk, recognizing the importance of this subject. The price of access was anonymity, and identifying details have been changed. Anonymity prevented me from writing more fully about how care sits in a geography of relationship. As more of our lives move online, instantly available on a screen or from Alexa, care remains offline, because so much of it relates to physical presence and touch: bathing, feeding, cleaning, tidying, holding a hand, observation, to name a few. Proximity can become critical: who lives near enough to drop by, to bring food or offer company. Across the country, the availability of care is unevenly spread; the gaps can be particularly acute, for example, in some rural and coastal areas with large elderly populations, or for single mothers with small children in an unfamiliar neighbourhood. Providing care can never be an individual responsibility; it is set in a web of who knows who nearby, how they meet and what relationships they develop. Decades of increasing geographical mobility have eroded many of the community networks vital to the provision of care in the past.

Delving into care has been a journey of discovery and personal reckoning. I have lived this book more intensely than any other; I was doing what I was writing about and I found myself bouncing between research and the need to provide care. I bring to the subject my life experience as mother and daughter, friend and sister, a few stints as a volunteer, and an expectation that there is much more to learn about care in the years ahead. But care has never been part of my professional life. For these interviews, I was an outsider looking into worlds I knew little about. I asked questions and heard a wide range of different heartfelt answers.

I learnt how care need not be gendered, and how it can all too easily be crushed in false dualisms, such as head/heart, active/passive or skilled/unskilled. Good care is as much an art as a skill, as much competence as tact. The highly qualified doctor is as capable of developing the capacity to care as the female homecare worker with few qualifications. I learnt that care can never be standardized – that's part of its current crisis; it is full of the unpredictable, the spontaneous, and the intensely personal. In interviews or at the back of meetings, I felt tears prick my eyes, and on occasion had to pause my questions when people were overcome recounting their experiences. Care may often be routine, but unexpected and powerful significance can be wrapped into small details – the raw stuff which gives people dignity and meaning in their lives, for both caregiver and recipient. My research proved humbling beyond anything I had ever imagined. It felt *important*, as I faced squarely a set of issues which our society has become adept at tucking out of sight.

As I look to the future, I think of what my daughter and sons might need to know; what painful surprises I can hope to warn them of, even prepare them for, and what rich rewards may arrive to inspire them. I would start by offering them this working definition: care runs through a range of human relationships which, while very differently constituted, deal with vulnerability, dependence and suffering. However reluctant we may be to face up to these three, they will inevitably form part of our life experience. Everybody has reason to nourish a culture's traditions of care. Our lives will depend on it, and already do in many more ways than we can begin to grasp.

I

The Invisible Heart

*'We humanize what is going on in the world
and in ourselves only by speaking of it, and
in the course of speaking of it we learn to be
human.'*

HANNAH ARENDT, *Men in Dark Times*, 1968

On a crisp autumn day with the sunlight catching the last of the leaves, I watched a group of small children walking in the park. They were about three years old and I counted eight of them. They were wearing high-vis green tabards, and were accompanied by two nursery staff. Forming a tight crocodile, they walked in pairs. As I looked more closely I saw that they were strapped by their wrists to each other, and to those in front and behind. The staff had to keep directing them forward for fear that if one stumbled, they would all come down. Their leader called out in a cheery voice, drawing their attention to a circle on a signpost here, a square there, eager to improve their recognition of geometrical shapes. The children anxiously jostled in their close formation, trying to avoid tripping over each other.

Such encounters are routine in my local park, and deeply

jarring. Children of that age want to wander, stop, go backwards or even around in circles; they want to explore and experiment. This is childcare of the most regimented (literally) kind, with parallels closer to incarceration than to the spontaneity or freedom essential to play. What are we forgetting? How can tying children up, or ratios of four small children per adult, be an acceptable form of care?

When we are catapulted by emergency into depending on the care of others, we are acutely aware of its quality: at a moment of anxiety, we may deeply value the gentle humour of a paramedic, the attentiveness of a nurse or the kindliness of a doctor. When these are absent and staff are harassed, impatient or unavailable, we sense the fraying of the fabric of care on which we rely. Care underpins so many aspects of our lives that its many manifestations can obscure the commonalities between childcare, healthcare and care of the elderly. When we take notice, we see care shifting to something unrecognizable, inimical to human flourishing. Just as haunting as that crocodile of small children is the care home on my way to the bus stop; I've passed it a thousand times or more and never seen a soul in the garden, never seen a window open or the thick net curtains pulled back to allow in the sunshine. Like care homes up and down the country, it is a world separate to itself, secret and introverted, where the elderly sit and wait.

The care crisis is one of culture, politics and ethics in the face of dramatic social change. A deep-seated historical prejudice against the value and importance of care is colliding with twenty-first-century lives. The crisis has two dimensions: care is either unavailable and gaps are opening up, or its quality is deeply compromised. As I visited homes, hospitals, GP surgeries, care agencies, care homes and hospices, common themes emerged from snatched conversations between appointments, or over a hurried sandwich in staff rooms and cluttered offices.

The need for care is increasing in several distinct ways. One well-known cause is demographic change; between 2001 and 2015, the number of people over eighty-five increased by 38 per cent, and it will double between 2016 and 2041. On average, the last six years of these longer lives are accompanied by acute frailty, multiple medications and a complex round of medical appointments, usually in addition to the traditional tasks of feeding, bathing and assistance with the toilet. The medical journal *The Lancet* projects that the number of over eighty-fives requiring twenty-four-hour care will double by 2035. There is no evidence of society creating the sustainable structures – institutions, policies, sources of funding – to meet this historically unprecedented challenge.

The issue of who cares for the elderly is caught between powerful expectations: on the one hand that the family should meet the need, and on the other that the welfare state is responsible, with its historic ambition of care from 'cradle to grave'. But neither the average family nor the state was ever expected to meet this type of care; in 1908, when provision of a state pension first passed into law, life expectancy was forty-seven for men and fifty for women. The nineteenth-century novelist's romantic image of the loving daughter caring for her parents was the exception, as so many women died in childbirth. Historical surveys reveal that in the UK, households rarely incorporated more than two generations: the 'granny in the corner' is a myth. The family often couldn't or didn't cope, and the brutal nineteenth-century workhouse system, intended to deal with the idle and work-shy, tragically filled up with the elderly. Significantly, the advent of the welfare state did not lead immediately to an improvement in the care of the elderly; through the 1960s and 1970s, the scandal of the crowded hospital 'back wards' stirred the public conscience. We are again in danger of a mismatch of provision and need as the elderly are caught in a cycle of hospital stays.

Care for the elderly is putting huge pressure on families. The bulk is provided by partners, themselves often elderly; 1.3 million people in England and Wales aged sixty-five and over are carers, and their numbers are rising fast. Typically, wives care for their husbands, but husbands also become carers. Between the age of seventy-five and eighty-four, carers have gender parity; above eighty-five, it is men who form the majority (58 per cent to 41 per cent women). Next in line to provide care are the offspring in their fifties and sixties, and their numbers are stepping up dramatically: between 2001 and 2015 there was a 16.5 per cent increase in carers in this age group. Over the same period, the hours of care provided also rose, with a 33 per cent increase in those offering fifty hours or more per week, and a 43 per cent increase in those providing twenty to forty-nine hours. Some research claims that over a third of carers find their tasks take up more than 100 hours a week; this is a group in desperate need of support. Much of this need is met by women; one in four women in their fifties and sixties are carers, twice the number of men of the same age, and one third of these women have multiple care responsibilities. Women of this age group face years of care for parents and then partners in their mid to later years, an experience which was rare amongst their predecessors. It has been estimated that 1.7 million women have had to leave work to care for family members, many because they feel the alternatives are either too expensive or of poor quality.

Another reason the need for care is growing is the number of people with a long-term health condition: the figure increased by 16 per cent between 2001 and 2015, and now totals 12 million people. Survival rates for major illnesses such as cancer and strokes have improved, while diseases such as diabetes and dementia are sharply on the rise. In addition, hospitals are pressured to speed up the discharge of patients, leaving the task of caring for the convalescent to family. The cottage hospital has largely disappeared. People with disabilities are living longer – something to celebrate as a remarkable achievement of medical science, but less consideration has been given to how these longer lives are to be supported and enjoyed. Convalescents, the long-term ill and people with disabilities, all with needs which were once met by institutions under the supervision of medical professionals, now rely on family carers. At the same time, the shape of families has changed; the 'beanpole' family is stretched across generations and often geographically scattered. As social scientist David Halpern points out, 'the consequence is that risks have become much more concentrated and potentially more devastating. In a large extended family, if one person is sick the burden is spread out; in a household of three or four – or even of one – it's a massive and catastrophic burden.'

Historically the assumption was that the women of the family would provide care, an assumption which proves powerfully persistent. Yet it comes into conflict with a salient fact of twenty-first-century Britain: women's employment rates are at an all-time high of 78 per cent. Women who may once have been available to care for the elderly or sick are now at work. Women's employment has been welcomed by employers as flexible and cheap, and for most women work has been a hard-won chance to gain financial independence, status and relief from domestic isolation. The proportion of mothers with pre-school-age children in paid work has grown from less than a half to two thirds in the last twenty years, as governments of left and right have encouraged women back into employment to increase household income and reduce the reliance of single parents on the state. However, they have not matched that enthusiasm with investment in care. They have relied on women to take on the so-called double shift – paid work and care.

The state has been markedly reluctant to meet the need for childcare. After piecemeal initiatives, it was only in 1998 that the government offered to fund a meagre 12.5 hours of free care for four-year-olds – merely a token gesture. It was not until 2017, nearly twenty years later, that government provision reached thirty hours of free care for three- and four-year-olds. Childcare for under-threes remains the most expensive in Europe, accounting for 40 per cent of disposable family income. Grandparents are an essential lifeline for those lucky enough to have them nearby; nine million offer an average of eight hours care a week. One in four families depends on them, saving families £16 billion a year in childcare costs. William Beveridge, the great architect of the welfare state in the 1940s, assumed – as have many succeeding politicians – that women would continue to rock the cradle. The result is a makeshift childcare system in which provision is dogged by chronic underfunding, leading to dangerous compromises on quality. Here is another dimension of the crisis of care.

The difficulties of parents juggling shifts, finding after-school clubs and breakfast clubs, and latchkey kids looking after younger siblings have become the everyday routine in UK families, a system easily thrown by a detail going awry, such as a case of flu or a doctor's appointment. Family life has precariousness built in, analogous to the 'just-in-time' model of supermarkets and manufacturers, designed to cut the cost of holding stock so the materials are only shipped when needed. Household finances are now usually based on the model of two earners; there is little capacity to deal with the unpredictable, and time and energy to support other relatives, let alone neighbours, is scarce. As people's working lives extend into their late sixties, grandparents also have to juggle childcare with their jobs. Inherently fragile, these patterns generate anxiety not just in the family but in the wider community. It marks a significant change from a past when women developed support networks to share the unpredictable and sometimes overwhelming care needs in many working-class communities. The communal care infrastructure, famously described by Michael Young and Peter Willmott in their influential book *Family and Kinship in East London* in the 1950s, has largely disappeared.

Another dimension adds strain to the care responsibilities within the family. Parenting has become a longer process, with children dependent – financially and, often, emotionally – until well into their twenties. High housing costs are producing a new family structure in which young adults live at home into their late twenties or longer (1999–2014 saw a 46 per cent increase in the numbers of young people aged eighteen to twenty-four living at home). Such multigenerational households were the exception in the past, when parents usually regarded their responsibility to provide as finite; teenage girls and boys were routinely sent into service or apprenticeships, expected to pay their way or contribute to the household tasks of caring for younger siblings. In 1900 the parental care of providing board and lodging may have lasted for only twelve or fifteen years – emotional ties, of course, lasting longer – whereas now parenting is often a twenty-five-year project, as young people's independence and 'settling down' becomes ever more uncertain and provisional. Over the last sixty years, the parental role has also become more complex. High expectations fall on parents, not just to provide basics such as food and shelter, but also to develop strong emotional bonds. The authoritarian model of parenting has been replaced by one of close emotional intimacy and shared leisure time. Washing machines and ready-made meals may have eased the physical aspects of care, but the emotional demands have increased, and the parent – usually the mother – is expected to empathize, intuit and provide solidarity during the long maturation to adulthood.

Much of this can be deeply rewarding and enriching for both parent and offspring, but it represents an intensification of parenting, and can add to the strain of juggling home and work. An increase in mental ill health amongst young people has exacerbated the pressure, requiring parents to help, support, safeguard and find a way through the lottery of treatment. For a parent struggling to hold down a job, the effort is exhausting, and, for some, beyond their capacity. When they look to public services for help, they are met by waiting lists and a rationing of overstretched services. For many women, caring is engrained in the definition of what it is to be a woman, a wife, a mother, sister and daughter. The impact of these growing needs for care of both young and old can provoke an anguished and often heroic effort to reconcile the impossible, and maintain traditions of care in a set of novel circumstances.

Yet the irony is that care as the responsibility of the nuclear family is a recent phenomenon dating from the second half of the twentieth century. Because the care needs of the very young and very old can be immensely demanding, families always looked beyond their immediate circle for help. Relatives were called upon, but even more significant was the army of women in domestic service; in 1931, domestic service was the largest source of employment for women, accounting for one in four of all women in paid work. The Downton Abbey image of footmen and parlour maids has obscured the more mundane reality: a general maid was regarded as essential in most households, and even in relatively poor families a girl helped out, minding children for a few hours. The shift of this large female workforce into factory, retail and clerical work after the Second World War was the first of the great waves of disinvestment in household care in the twentieth century, to be followed by wives and mothers going out to work a few decades later.

The 'servant problem' became an acute preoccupation for

middle-class women in the middle decades of the twentieth century as they found themselves expected to take over the task of looking after a family full time. As female paid employment rates climbed from the 1970s onwards, it was assumed that domestic life was manageable thanks to technological breakthroughs such as washing machines and dishwashers, or could be squeezed into evenings and weekends. That assumption was based on widespread ignorance about what women – paid and unpaid – had been doing with their time in the home in the first place. What lies at the heart of the crisis of care is a history of invisibility, which began in the home and family but now casts a long shadow over all care work.

The invisibility of care is evident through centuries of Western thought. The economist Adam Smith, who wrote *The Wealth of Nations* in 1776, based his ideas on 'homo economicus', viewing man as an independent agent calculating his self-interest in the market through cost-benefit analysis. Women played no part in his theory; they had no autonomy and were bound by dependence on their husbands, and by their children's dependence on them. The rationale for their role in the home was different to that of the market: they were motivated by self-denial rather than competition, sentiment not rationality, tenderness not calculation. The feminist economist Nancy Folbre argues that while men's activities at work were governed by the 'invisible hand' of the market, the corollary for women was the 'invisible heart'; 'care has been framed as instinctive, biological, natural and moral – so it's not work in the narrow sense as understood by eighteenth-century economists'.

In 1694 the remarkably outspoken Mary Astell, a self-educated merchant's daughter, questioned the division of labour between men and women: 'such generous offices we do them; such ungenerous returns they make us'. But such sharp-eyed observations were rare. Women were urged to regard their work as carers as a spiritual practice of patience, self-effacement and self-denial; they were expected to collude in the invisibility of caring, seen as a true and modest expression of femininity. Industrialization hardened the distinctions between the public world and the private, the different values of market and home, men and women. J. S. Mill wrote in *The Subjection of Women* that women 'are universally taught that they are born and created for self-sacrifice', and lamented 'the exaggerated self-abnegation which is the present artificial ideal of feminine character'. In *The American Woman's Home* (1869), Catherine Beecher and her sister Harriet Beecher Stowe advised that woman's 'great mission is self-denial'. Women were expected to care for their husbands, children, the sick and the elderly without complaint. It was their duty but also their salvation. As Folbre comments, 'patriarchy was not just a means of privileging men, it was also a means of ensuring an adequate supply of care'.

Home was to be 'the haven in a heartless world' and women were the 'angel of the house' according to nineteenth-century ideals; women were 'maintained as a redemptive counterpart to the world of capitalism', suggests the sociologist Sharon Hays. 'This intense idealization of women and home reflects a widespread ambivalence about the values of the market – the calculating behaviour of *homo economicus* – and impersonal bureaucracy.' According to theories of capitalism, everything and everyone had a price, and this was articulated as a rational and impersonal truth, and defended as progress. But this market paradigm provoked unease because of its brutal inhumanity and the suffering it caused – workers thrown out of jobs or children working long hours in factories. Furthermore, it offered a chilling prescription for intimate human relationships, and had to be specifically excluded from the private world of family life. As industrial capitalism increased its hold on society, aspects of private life were shielded. The expanding middle classes enthusiastically reinvented the meaning of family and home. Marriage was no longer regarded as primarily a practical arrangement expanding property and family connections, but as a relationship in which the angelic wife offered succour and tenderness. Similarly, childhood came to be seen as a time of enchantment, innocence and delight. Both were reimagined (the reality was another matter) to express the experiences, emotions and relationships no longer acceptable in the male world of the capitalist economy.

Separate spheres confined the sexes to rigidly defined roles, from which women – and some men – struggled to escape. This idealization bore little relationship to the working lives of millions of working-class women, and for middle-class women, it was underpinned by the cheap labour of domestic servants and the suppression of any aspiration to independence. The idealization was famously described by Coventry Patmore in his narrative poem 'The Angel in the House', first published in 1854. Virginia Woolf subjected the notion to scornful disdain in her satirical essay 'Professions for Women': 'The Angel in the House ... was immensely charming. She was utterly unselfish. She excelled in the difficult arts of family life. She sacrificed herself daily. If there was chicken, she took the leg; if there was a draught, she sat in it.' Woolf wanted to murder her: 'I acted in self-defence. Had I not killed her she would have killed me ... She was always creeping back when I thought I had despatched her.'

But the Angel of the House proved more persistent than even Woolf could have imagined, and she still hovers over expectations of care work, both paid and unpaid. In 1982 the feminist Wendy Whitfield recounted in *Spare Rib* how she went on strike: 'I would do only *my* shopping, cooking and cleaning ... I would not clean up nor would I keep up my incessant tidying, writing of lists, washing and returning of milk bottles, putting away of dishes that he left to drain instead of drying them, defrosting the fridge or cleaning the cooker, clearing away the coffee cups or writing to his relatives ... It is up to us to remember that men are conditioned to expect servicing.' Nearly forty years on, Whitfield's declaration is still relevant. Despite the huge increase of women in paid work, they do around sixteen hours of housework a week compared to men's six. The difference is even more stark in other countries: in Portugal, women do five hours, twenty-eight minutes a day compared to men's one hour, thirty-six minutes.

What eighteenth-century economists overlooked was that Aristotle's original definition of the term 'economics' was derived from *oikos*, meaning household. In *Politics*, he considered both the paid labour of the husband and the household duties of the wife, but in succeeding centuries the latter was ignored by philosophers and economists. The struggle for feminists in recent decades has been to make good this glaring omission. Virginia Held, a pioneering philosopher of care, urges that 'for limited purposes we may imagine each other as liberal individuals in the marketplace, independent, autonomous and rational ... but we should not lose sight of the deeper reality of human interdependency and of the need for caring relations to undergird or surround such constructions. The artificial abstraction of the model of the liberal individual is at best suitable for a restricted and limited part of human life, rather than the whole of it.' Held advocates an ethics of care in which emotion and the capacity to build relationship are valued. 'Sympathy, empathy, sensitivity and responsiveness are seen as the kind of moral emotions that need to be cultivated, even anger might be a component. This is not about raw emotion, they still need to be reflected on and educated.' Held reminds us that 'many of our responsibilities are not freely entered into but presented to us by the accidents of our embeddedness in familial and social and historical contexts. It often calls on us to *take* responsibility while liberal individualist morality focuses on how we should leave each other alone.'

A vivid illustration of the invisibility of care was the work of the vast army of servants – one of the overlooked antecedents of care work such as nursing and social care. Servants left behind little record of their lives, and have been neglected by historians. Despite being the largest source of female employment until well into the twentieth century, the subject warrants only three mentions in E. P. Thompson's *The Making of the English Working Class*. Servants were literally ignored: middle-class homes had separate entrances, staircases and living quarters. In some households, servants were expected to go to elaborate lengths to conceal their presence; they had to face the wall or withdraw behind a door to avoid encountering a master or mistress. Maids were advised to wear non-creaking shoes, and encouraged to move quietly. Servants usually entered rooms without knocking and their arrival with trays or additional coals was unacknowledged. The novelist G. K. Chesterton, reflecting on his middle-class childhood, admitted that his home knew 'far too little of its own servants' and that hanging over the subject was 'a sort of silence and embarrassment'. A Prussian commentator admired how English servants were 'so entirely excluded from all familiarity, and such profound respect is exacted from them, that they appear to be considered rather as machines than as beings of the same order'. Servants worked exceptionally long hours, rising early to light fires, their days filled with a round of endless work before retiring to bed late. In 1853 the manual *Common Sense for Housemaids* proposed that 'a really good housemaid should never be able to be alone in a room with a table without giving it a good rub, or, if the room is occupied, without wishing to do so'. Mrs Miniver, the fictional author of a popular column in *The Times* in the 1930s, wrote that housework should be the 'low, distant humming in the background'.

As servants moved into new forms of employment in the twentieth century, their work fell to their former mistresses, but the cultural value of it remained meagre. 'Women's work' was a term of denigration. This history continues to affect the cultural value of care, and is one reason why care is persistently regarded as unskilled work and is expected to be free or cheap. Care work is routinely belittled and dismissed, even by those doing it. Repeatedly, care workers I spoke with struggled to explain the value of their work; they referred to their low status with comments such as, 'I'm just a carer,' and recounted anecdotes of slights they had received.

Yet care work is the fastest-growing employment sector in industrialized societies and represents 13 per cent of all jobs in the UK, the single largest source of employment. When attempts are made to put a monetary value on unpaid care, the figures are dizzying. In 1995 the United Nations costed the work of unpaid carers throughout the world – caring for the young, sick, and elderly – at about 16 trillion dollars; it admitted that even this huge figure could be an underestimate and that 'household nonmarket activity' could be the equivalent of 80 per cent of the gross world product. More recently, unpaid care (often referred to as 'informal care') in the UK was valued at £59.5 billion by the Office of National Statistics. The consensus is that care work represents a half to a third of GDP in every country. In 2015 a team valued just the unpaid work of carers for the sick and elderly at £132 billion a year, more than the value of HSBC holdings, and close to the annual cost of the NHS. Carers were saving the public purse £2.5 billion a week, or £362 million a day, or £15.1 million an hour. By the time it takes you to read a few of these chapters, unpaid carers will have saved the state millions. The scale of this voluntary care service, upon which the NHS depends, is growing all the time, yet it is rarely acknowledged, and the only financial support – the Carer's Allowance – is the lowest state benefit available.

Capitalism was built on ignoring and marginalizing the care work of women. This much has been the history of centuries, but a further insidious shift has taken place in the last few decades, as market principles have been introduced into the care relationships from which they were once explicitly excluded. We have 'begun to think and define ourselves and everything else in terms of market values', warns the philosopher Michael Sandel. He points out how monetary terms crowd out other meanings, such as ethical and political considerations; the person involved is lost to sight, and what was seen as a vocation is commodified as purely an employment contract. The result is that a set of cultural contradictions are now endemic in many forms of care work. The market depends on measurement so that it can analyse efficiency, productivity and competitiveness. To apply this to care requires redefining it as a series of tasks with specified outputs and then allocating those tasks to the lowest level of skill possible. The model is that developed for the manufacture of Ford cars in the early twentieth century by the management theorist Frederick Taylor.

Alison Leary, Professor of Healthcare at South Bank University, argues it is inappropriate for care: 'The Taylor model gives the false illusion of control and predictability. It works with biscuits and cars but not healthcare, where it becomes positively dangerous. The problem is that while you can teach a low-skill person how to do a repetitive task, it takes a lot of education and skill to cope with all the possible outcomes and be alert to spot them. Nursing, for example, is stochastic – a mathematical term – in which systems and processes change in a random way. Nursing is not deterministic, whereby one thing can be reliably predicted to produce a certain outcome. In healthcare, every process produces lots of different probabilities, like a firework going off in different directions. You can't predict all the outcomes from all the variables.' Leary gave an example of a unit where a central line had to be inserted for administering chemotherapy. 'The line can go straight into the heart and you need to use radiation to put it in. In our study, a team of nurses were doing it all day, every day, and were good at keeping patients calm, so there was no need for sedation. But a manager concluded that it was a routine thing and could be done by someone of lower skill. But one of the possible side effects is a collapsed lung, which is very serious. A nurse would know what to do in that situation. You need a high degree of discriminative judgement to manage such risks.'

In another study, Leary was trying to calculate optimal workload: 'We found the priority people focused on were the tasks, and technical work such as drugs rounds. What got left undone was relationship, communication, and giving the patient information.' Yet these three are crucial to the patient's care.

Individual care workers are expected to reconcile market principles with their own understanding of people's needs and their responsibility, and interviewees often spoke of the struggle to manage the resulting contradictions. Putting prices on items in a hospital store cupboard or on a vaccination in a GP surgery may seem a small detail, but it is a significant and pervasive ideological reframing inserted into everyday routines: flags have been planted across the territory, introducing commodification into healthcare so that actions, conversations and medical procedures take on a monetary value.

Advertising brings more contradictions, by raising expectations. On one of my research trips when I was shadowing nurses, I noticed every day on my way into the hospital a prominently placed advert by the main entrance: 'Care in your home, the way you want it.' Care has become a thing, subject to the consumer's desires, and available as part of a monetary transaction. As a nurse explained in an interview: 'There is a confusion between want and need, and that is how consumerism works: it turns wants into the imperative of needs.' The care system is overloaded as needs become demands, and essential dimensions of the relationship between carer and recipient are hidden or lost altogether – such as reciprocity, and the carer's autonomy over how to engage their heart in the work as well as their hands and head.

That prominently placed poster was playing its part, shaping the expectations and understanding of all the staff, patients and visitors entering the hospital. In a coffee break on the ward, a nurse talked to me resentfully of a 'culture of entitlement', and complained that some patients even clicked their fingers for attention. Patients are asked to rate their experience of GP appointments in the same way they rate a flight, shifting the nature of the encounter to that of a consumer contract. The ubiquitous use of the verb 'deliver' in the language of health and social care is problematic: you can deliver parcels or fast food; you can't deliver a relationship. 'To deliver' is to hand over something, but care is rarely so finite or so tightly circumscribed; it is too often tangled up with intimacy and vulnerability.

Concepts of consumerism were enthusiastically introduced by the New Labour governments of the 2000s into public services such as health and education. Looking back in 2019, the writer Will Davies perceptively argued that 'Blair's gambit was that only by keeping pace with the expectations of an increasingly consumerist culture could public services retain credibility and support. This may have been true in the medium term, but it eventually leaves the public sector without any justification or cultural identity of its own. It is a state-led strategy for hollowing out and talking down public services (as distinct from business), even as New Labour was pouring unprecedented sums of money into public services.'

Health and social-care staff are caught in the crossfire between this creeping commercialization and their intuitive understanding of care as a relationship requiring qualities which can't be bought or sold. I observed that it was those at the bottom of institutional hierarchies who felt the contradiction keenly, and they developed their own forms of resistance – grumbling, complaining or dogged persistence – as they stubbornly held on to their personal values. Even at senior levels, I met those troubled by how the commercial reframing shifts the ground under everyone's feet. A director of nursing admitted she describes nursing as a 'business', and uses arguments about cost savings to make the case for more investment in nursing. 'I have to put a financial value on care. I argue that better care costs more but saves money in the long run. To do that, I have to make the business case for nursing, but the use of these words brings a danger of commercializing something which is not commercial. Does everything at this hospital have to have a monetary value? Of course not.' She went on to elaborate a definition of care as a form of ethical development: 'The skill of caring is acquired through a learning journey, as you learn about yourself, and others. The most important thing in a nurse is a sense of humanity. They need to be accepting of difference, and have a regard and curiosity about people. Kindness is so important.'

She was switching between multiple framings for care: was it a business, a matter of saving money or an understanding of shared humanity? These are profoundly different forms of human activity. The management ethos of competition, drive, goals and focus may be appropriate in a commercial context, but often in care it produces too narrow a field of attention. Generating anxiety and stress, it can squeeze the capacity for those more expansive, expressive qualities such as kindness and compassion.

It is no surprise that feminism defined itself in opposition to care, given its low status and invisibility. Simone De Beauvoir was vehement, describing the drudgery of motherhood as 'absurd vegetation'. She railed against women's domesticity in *The Second Sex*: 'few tasks are more like the torture of Sisyphus than housework with its endless repetition. The clean becomes soiled, the soiled is made clean, over and over, day after day.' She analysed how the 'intimate relationship between caring and femininity is how one sex is differentiated from the other ... [for women] caring is the defining characteristic of their self-identity and their life's work. Not caring becomes the defining characteristic of male identity.'

The Second Sex was published in 1949, just as middle-class women were having to fill the gap left by their departing servants. In 1957 Betty Friedan wrote in *The Feminine Mystique*, 'the problem lay buried, unspoken. It was a strange stirring, a sense of dissatisfaction, a yearning ... As she made the beds, shopped for groceries, she was afraid to ask even of herself the silent question – "Is this all?"' These books became the manifestos of second-wave feminism, inspiring women to a life beyond the family and home. In 1971 Margaret Adams argued that the defining of femininity as care had locked women into 'self-defeating trivialities' depriving society of women's contribution.

It was a form of feminism which sank deep into my soul. I remember as a child my fascination with the cover of one of my mother's books: an image of a women struggling to burst out from the roof of her house, trapped by a net. It intrigued and horrified me. This new feminism set its sights on the world of paid work and careers, eager to assert a new female independence and autonomy. Arriving in the US in the mid-1980s, I spotted a cigarette advert which encapsulated my generation's aspirations: 'You've come a long way,' read the slogan above the image of a sharply dressed, beautiful woman superimposed on a sepia photo of her forebears, bent double scrubbing floors. Women set off to work, convinced that it was only a failure of willpower that allowed the highest echelons of every career to be dominated by men. Even when children arrived, many women were expected to be back at their desks within a few months of the baby's birth. By the early 1990s, with unprecedented numbers of women in employment, some even argued that the task of feminism was done. Others were honest enough to admit to feeling exhausted. The shift of women into paid work was not matched by men taking up more domestic tasks. 'Having it all' became a phrase to beat women with: the implication was that they were deluding themselves that they could have both family life and work, and they were bringing the ensuing difficulties of juggling and overstretch on themselves.

In the mid-1990s Maureen Freely was astute enough to call it out: motherhood had been abandoned by feminists. Those who were fifteen years older had been determined to break out of the domestic trap, and those fifteen years younger had moved their focus to questions of sexualization and identity. Mothers in the 1990s had been parked in a lay-by, Freely suggested; women were workers first and mothers second, if at all. Motherhood had become a hobby – a task requiring much larger resources of time and energy had been relegated to women's spare time. The liberal feminism of the 1980s may have opened up women's horizons, but it stripped bare the unpaid care economy, leaving significant gaps; women were left to find their own solutions, and were blamed when they failed. The only way to resolve this dilemma, argued socialist feminism, was to recognize and value women's unpaid care work (the Wages for Housework campaign was one expression of this argument) and to ensure comprehensive public provision as the essential precondition of women's freedom. Early advocates such as Dora Russell and Sylvia Pankhurst had argued that childbearing was central to women's lives and should not be subordinated to their economic role. But by the 1980s this vision of collective action and a generous welfare state survived only on the margins of British politics.

The model of two working parents was an intimidating experiment, and many either chose not to join it, or did not find a partner interested in doing so. Childlessness has nearly doubled; 18 per cent of women aged forty-five in 2017 were childless, compared to 10 per cent of the generation born in 1945. An unprecedented proportion of women will reach old age without the support of children, generating new demands for care outside the family.

Feminism has forged ahead in recent years on many fronts, but a recognition and valuing of care is noticeably absent. The pay gap and the lack of women in senior positions routinely prompt outrage, but the undervaluing and invisibility of care is a major driver of both. The focus of activism remains firmly fixed on achievement, self-expression, identity and image rather than the work of care which dominates so many women's lives.

Nor have we begun to reckon with a more pervasive and intangible loss of how women maintained a set of values (often at their own cost) in human relationships. As the sociologist Angela McRobbie put it in a BBC interview in 2006: 'There has been a marked shift away from what feminists used to call the "ethic of care". It was a defining feature of women's lives – caring for others, caring for children, elderly people, community. It stands to reason that as women enter the labour market, their time is going to be limited for caring. The easy answer is to say that caring rightly has become a profession in its own right, and there's a lot of sense to that. On the other hand, we all know the debate about wider values that accrue to giving care in society.

If that's replaced by ruthless individualism, by straightforward competitiveness, then it's a toxic brew.' At a conference on care, one nurse echoed McRobbie's concern, arguing that the lack of understanding of care amounted to a suppression of what she described as the 'feminine principle' in our culture. She defined the latter as 'a principle which doesn't seek perfection or power but fosters human connection, nurturing and compassion'. Virginia Held warns in *The Ethics of Care* that 'if women in their justifiable quest for equality pursue justice at the expense of care, morality will suffer. For those previously engaged in care to become more and more like the free and equal, rational and unencumbered individuals of theories of justice will leave no one to nurture the relations of family and friendship, and to cultivate the ties of caring.'

Forced to accommodate the capitalist system, feminism made a Faustian bargain: women gained a degree of freedom, but at the cost of privatizing the ethic of care, turning it into an accident of character or personal preference, rather than the fundamental basis on which human well-being rests. Eager to prove their worth in the workplace, feminists were unable to claim the time and space for care, forced to squeeze it around the demands of the job. Meanwhile not enough men rallied to the task and a new distribution of care. A social revolution left the job half done.

The failure of our society to recognize care has its roots in these historical trends, but since 2010 the dismantling of key parts of the welfare state has made the situation acute. A precarious and unsustainable combination of rising female employment, increasing need for care, and inadequate public services has collided with a decade of painful cuts following the global financial crash of 2008. The policy of austerity has included holding down the pay of those working in care-related jobs. From social care to childcare and nursing, the largely female workforce has been expected to bear the brunt of austerity in their pay packets. Yet again, cultural stereotypes have re-emerged, assuming that care should be cheap.

Local authorities have suffered some of the worst cuts: central-government funding halved between 2010 and 2018, leading to a cut of 8 per cent in social-care budgets at a time when demand was growing from an ageing population (as a comparison, NHS budgets increased at 9 per cent to meet growing need over the same period). Local authorities made savings in two ways: by tightening the criteria for care – it is estimated that around 1.4 million elderly people who would have been eligible for care now fall outside any state provision – and by holding costs down on care contracts, which, in turn, brought down wages. Only one in seven local authorities pay care providers the price regarded as necessary to comply with minimum employment standards and ensure sustainability of the sector.

The result has been endemic low pay across the workforce of 1.47 million social carers, with a persistent problem of pay below the minimum wage (estimated to affect up to 220,000 workers), widespread use of zero-hours contracts and no payment for travel time. The system is chronically underfunded. Enforcement of employment law is ineffective, with minimal inspections; in 2017/8 HMRC prosecuted only eighty employers for illegal underpayment, out of a total of 21,200 providers, representing just 0.3 per cent. Research in 2011 estimated that 9–13 per cent of care jobs, employing 157,000–219,000 workers, were paid below the minimum wage; more up-to-date figures are likely to be higher as the cuts have continued to grip social-care budgets. Increasing pay to minimum levels compliant with the law would threaten the entire system. Tellingly, a recent court decision that employees working shifts which require staying the night (known as sleep-in shifts) should be paid the

minimum wage led HMRC to suspend its enforcement, fearful
that the cost of paying arrears and future costs 'would threaten
the stability and long-term viability of providers'. (The court
decision was overturned and is now subject to appeal.) The
financial precariousness and importance of the sector puts it
beyond the reach of the law.

This pattern of chronic low pay has led to high turnover and
vacancy rates. Every year nearly half of care workers leave their
job. This churn rate is disastrous, as continuity and experience
are lost and resources are diverted to constant recruitment
efforts. It is evidence of how the work can provoke deep distress; in March 2017 a study of suicide trends found that the rate
amongst care workers is twice the national average. Increasingly
providers claim they cannot find staff; vacancy rates ran at 7.8
per cent in 2019, a total of 122,000 unfilled jobs, twice the rate
for the economy as a whole. The future of this workforce looks
bleak; it is ageing dramatically as young people look elsewhere
for work, and the average age has jumped to forty-seven in
recent years.

Historically, Britain has always imported care workers from
Ireland, the Caribbean, the Commonwealth and the EU, but
political resistance to migration chokes off this supply. By 2028,
a shortfall of 400,000 is predicted in the social-care workforce –
and that would only keep the system at its current, inadequate
level of provision. Yet none of this alarming picture provokes the
kind of engaged public concern which could force the government to act. An Ipsos Mori poll in 2019 highlighted this public
indifference: 87 per cent thought the NHS should be protected
from cuts; only 34 per cent thought social care should be (a
decline of nearly 10 per cent since 2015). The NHS continues
to dominate political attention, despite innumerable inquiries
urging action to improve social care to prevent the knock-on
impact on NHS beds and resources.

Nurses were also badly affected by the wage-freeze of austerity. By 2018 a starter nurse earned £23,000, an 8 per cent fall in pay after inflation since 2010. The result was a vacancy rate of about 10 per cent, with a turnover rate in 2018 that was 20 per cent higher than in 2012; more nurses are leaving the profession's register than are joining. With a sharp drop in applications from the European Union, the House of Commons Health Select Committee urged in 2018 that the nursing workforce be 'expanded at scale and pace' to meet the growing demand for care in the NHS. They warned that nurses were overstretched and struggling to cope with 'relentless pressures' and were expressing real anxiety about how to maintain accepted professional standards in such circumstances. The committee also warned that it will be difficult for the UK to recruit abroad when other countries are offering better pay and training.

The worst levels of pay have been in the childcare sector, where it is estimated that in 2018 40 per cent of staff were underpaid, the highest rate of underpayment in any sector 'by far', according to the Low Pay Commission. In 2017 a nursery manager's pay averaged £13.43 per hour, compared to £20.62 for equivalent occupations, while a childcare worker's pay was just £8.49 an hour. Despite low pay, overtime is frequently required (as much as 81 per cent of the workforce said they had been expected to put in extra hours according to a 2018 survey). Inevitably, low pay has led to persistent recruitment and retention issues across the sector, comparable to those in social care, adding stress to the task of managers already struggling with the large volumes of bureaucracy required to meet new standards for child development and with helping parents navigate complex funding systems.

The gap in funding the childcare system was estimated at £662 million in 2019 by experts, and has led to compromises on quality, with fewer trained staff and poorer staff–child ratios – an outcome which the Department of Education appeared to encourage when it advised that 'hourly costs can be reduced where providers deploy staff efficiently within statutory limits'. As one early-years expert, Sue Cowley, commented in her blog, 'The problem with looking at childcare in this way is that it ignores the realities of the sector, and even worse, it ignores the human beings working in it.' Some extra capacity in staffing is essential, she explained, to cope with the unexpected, such as illness. Ratios of carers to children have been raised to a level which many believe seriously compromises quality; one adult can care for six toddlers aged two, or four babies under one. The ratio can rise to thirteen three-year-olds to one adult in teacher-led nurseries. This is dangerous care on the cheap, and loses sight of its central purpose of child development. Care is being used as a way of warehousing children to ensure their mothers are available for paid work. One report ended on a note of suppressed panic, begging for increased investment, proper training and a 'universal change in the way society thinks about, and values, early-years education and childcare'.

During the many conversations I had with care workers, the influence of grandparents and parents hovered in the wings. An understanding of care work was often attributed to their example. The older generation was a source of inspiration and represented a palpable sense of continuity, a relay race in which the task of care was passed like a baton from parent to child, and, in time, from child back to parent. Often, this understanding expanded into concepts of service dedicated to the well-being of others, kindness to strangers and forms of solidarity. Interviewees would say, 'There but for the grace of God go I,' or mentioned the Golden Rule: 'Do unto others as you would have them do unto you.' Of the people I interviewed, a few of the care workers and several of those caring for their parents were religious, and their care was grounded in their faith, particularly amongst ethnic minorities. Many more mentioned that their parents and grandparents had been religious, but added that they were not; they still referred to elements of an ethical tradition which had inspired them and provided a sense of worth, yet which they felt was fading. Concepts they held dear, such as duty, kindliness and even responsibility, were disregarded by their employers and wider society.

Religion has played a major role in organizing care; hospitals began as religious institutions. All traditions urge the practice of compassion, an essential attribute of care. Secular humanism has incorporated much of this ethical practice, but religion approaches the task of educating and instilling ideals with repetitive reinforcement, determination and organization. Of course, religion is no guarantee of good care, and religious institutions have demonstrated appalling abuse of those in their care. But the impetus for reform and visionary expansion of provision have frequently sprung from religious inspiration. Take two pioneering figures whose influence is still evident today: both Florence Nightingale, a nurse in the Crimean war, and Beatrice Webb, an early advocate of the welfare state, were formed by their intense early experiences of religion and the injunctions to live out Christian compassion. Nightingale always framed her work within that context, while Webb moved to a political model, but Christianity was the starting point for firing their radical reimagining of who cares for whom, and how.

Nightingale (1820–1910) and Webb (1858–1943) were among the first women to benefit from access to education. They applied their learning to the Christian ethics and compassion that, as women, they were expected to exemplify, and took up new causes such as hospital reform and labour rights. They challenged complacency and indifference, marshalling what was needed – evidence, statistics, argument, celebrity myth, religious ideals – to advance their cause. They envisioned entirely new ways of organizing care. They took it out of the context of the private and the charitable to make it a matter of public concern requiring state action. They helped establish new professions of nursing and social work, opening them up to women and thus setting a pattern of employment which has persisted until today. An ideology entwining care, femininity and virtue ensured a plentiful and high-quality female workforce for nursing and teaching until the last decades of the twentieth century. As women moved into traditional male-dominated professions such as law, accountancy and management, commentators described it as the 'end of female altruism'. Alongside the increased opportunities for women, it also inadvertently contributed to the devaluing of care, with little consideration of how to inspire men to an equivalent widening of career choices to include care work.

As religion fades in Western societies, will secular humanism prove robust enough to defend the ideals which sustain care from the values of the market? The work of care becomes increasingly countercultural because it routinely requires forms of self-denial, setting aside one's own needs to meet another's. Care requires resistance to a dominant cultural preoccupation with the self – its image, desires and their fulfilment. Carers find themselves rebels in a culture which no longer promotes or validates their labours. Perhaps this is what provokes the references to grandparents or parents, or religious principle, as part of an effort to find a larger framing for their efforts. There has been a cultural orphaning of care as a vital human activity.

All this amounts to the crisis of care: long-term trends exacerbated by the withdrawal of state provision. Never properly understood or valued, care has lost even the status it once had, eroded by capitalism and austerity, and largely abandoned by liberal feminism. Those in care work, including those in the care professions, are required to work within structures which imitate market mechanisms. They are forced to justify themselves in terms of efficiency and productivity – market terms often inimical to the values intrinsic to offering care.

From the home to the labour market, the cultural significance of care, and the time, attention, presence and touch it entails, has gradually been stripped out. Even the most cursory of historical surveys demonstrates how practices of care are fragile cultural constructions, which are vulnerable to abuse because they deal with intimacy and dependence. But over the last century, there have been huge advances in Western democracies in ensuring high standards of care – for example in health care and the establishment of the welfare state; we have grown accustomed to them – we may even feel entitled to them – without fully acknowledging what it takes to sustain them in terms of recognition, funding, respect and value, from one generation to the next.

(i)

care

care, noun – 1. The provision of what is necessary for the health, welfare, maintenance and protection of someone or something. 2. Serious attention or consideration applied to doing something correctly or to avoid damage or risk. 3. A feeling of or occasion for anxiety.

care, verb – 1. Feel concern or interest; attach importance to something. 1.1 Feel affection or liking. 1.2 Like or be willing to do or have something. 2. Look after and provide for the needs of.

Care originates from the Old English word *caru*, meaning sorrow, anxiety, grief, and from the Old German word *chara*, meaning lament, or a burden of the mind. Another root is the Old Norse *kor*, for sickbed. Care has always been closely associated with suffering. Care entails a willingness to be present, to share grief, to remain steadfast in the face of life at its most painful, and deal with the messy physical reality of the body and its excretions. Virgil saw care as so burdensome that he placed the personified 'vengeful Cares' (*ultrices Curae*) before the entrance to the underworld. But the Latin *cura* combined this sense of burden with a more positive interpretation of attentiveness to another's welfare. Seneca saw care as the capacity which elevates humans to the level of the gods. Humans could achieve 'the good' through their powers of reasoning, but the good was 'perfected by care' he argued. The Stoics believed care was how we became fully human.

In a neglected Graeco-Roman myth, the goddess Care fashioned a human being out of mud, and asked Jupiter to give it the spirit of life. Terra insisted the being should bear her name, since it was made of earth. Saturn ruled that Jupiter would take back the being's soul after death, and Terra its body, but that, since Care had made this being, 'Let her have and hold it as long as it lives.' It would be called 'homo' – after *humus*, Latin for earth. Care 'has and holds' the human being, not in the sense of possession but of cherishing (as in Christian wedding vows), an acknowledgement that care sustains all lives.

The origins of the word 'care' combine two quite distinct ideas: care as a practical activity to support someone's welfare; and care as a matter of intention, thinking about someone with empathy, concern, even sorrow. The distinction is between caring *for* someone, and caring *about* them, shifting from action to intention and emotion. Often one cares about the person one is caring for – but not always; in paid care work this can be imprecise territory. Patients or an elderly person may want to be cared about as well as cared for, yet even the most dedicated nurse or care worker will struggle to care about all those under their charge. Ambiguity is written into care as it straddles ethics, practical action, thought and a set of emotional responses.

In his influential work *Being and Time*, the philosopher Martin Heidegger uses the word *Sorge*, 'care', to understand what it means to be human. *Sorge* is not just an attitude but a sensibility, a way of being in the world. Heidegger sees the human person as a constant process of multiple physical and emotional interactions with the environment. What drives these interactions is care. *Sorge* is how we engage with the world, pay attention and inevitably render ourselves vulnerable to anxiety and sorrow. Whatever you care about is subject to change, sickness, ageing and death. Paying attention cannot but bring you to a deeper awareness of this. The etymological root of *Sorge* is 'sorrow'. We have expressions such as 'careworn' and 'cares of the world' to reveal how weighty the demands of care can be. Influenced by Heidegger, the psychologist Erik Erikson placed care at the centre of his eight stages of the human life cycle. Adult caring was 'the generational task of cultivating strength in the next generation', and it may be 'parental, didactic, productive or curative'.

A review of the literature on nursing suggests the word 'care' was not used in the first half of the twentieth century. Since then it has become a central preoccupation in nursing and has replaced 'attending' to the sick, 'minding' children, and 'relief' of the elderly. It has spread to numerous aspects of welfare policy; care of the elderly, childcare, 'care in the community' are all examples of the application of this flexible word. 'Take care' is now a common substitute for 'goodbye', while 'caring' as an adjective describes pleasant, kindly characteristics in a person. A growing political and commercial lobby promotes 'self-care', using technology to manage and monitor our own health.

The use of the word in welfare policy, with its associations with dependence, has given rise to a critique from disability-rights activists, who have argued that care entails a power relationship, and the language must shift to one of rights and empowerment. Care is not always benign; it can be controlling and meddling.

A succession of feminist philosophers have sought to define the word. Joan Tronto sees care as a political as well as a moral concept: a form of work which includes 'everything that we do to maintain, continue and repair our world so that we can live in it as well as possible'. She picks out four ethical elements: attentiveness, responsibility, competence and responsiveness.

Sara Ruddick suggests that 'as much as care is labour, it is also relationship. Caring labour is intrinsically relational.' Rollo May insists that care is about more than emotion; it is 'about doing something, making decisions'. Some have suggested care is a virtue, but Virginia Held disagrees, arguing that it is not altruistic but 'a relation in which the carer and the cared for share an interest in mutual well being'.

2

Maintenance Art

*'Ethics are at the heart of care: how to deal
with dependency, vulnerability and trust, the
fragility and connectedness, the ever-recurring
problem of establishing boundaries between the
self and others.'*

SELMA SEVENHUIJSEN,
Citizenship and the Ethics of Care, 1998

Motherhood proved the training ground for most of what I know about care, and has prompted many of the questions which run through this book. I stumbled into my first definitions of care in the chaotic early years of small children, and have been learning ever since. To my shock, motherhood required a different way of being, and that entailed unlearning much of what I had understood adulthood to mean.

My daughter was born late one evening. After everyone left – her father, my sister, the midwife and obstetrician – I lay on one side, leaning over the edge of the bed, peering into the cot beside me and met Eleanor. 'Everyone' had not gone: there was now Eleanor. It was a night of wonder. I didn't sleep and neither did she. She gazed at me with big blue eyes which seemed full of knowledge and of deep, unfocused amazement. She seemed to have come from somewhere far away, and now here we were, two souls who had found themselves in this physical relationship of mother and daughter. All night I whispered to this knowing creature; it was a strange collection of bits of information that I thought she might need or want to know about the life she had arrived in. Later I joked that I had discussed 'affairs of state', describing political parties, governments, countries and the like. It felt like a discussion, not a monologue; those eyes seemed to understand, taking it all in, sizing up both me and the physical sensations of being alive. The light, the noise, the smells of a busy maternity ward. What is this? she seemed to be asking, and I tried to explain.

Morning came, we were discharged, and arrived home to the practicalities of caring for a newborn, breastfeeding and nappies. The sheer physicality of the relationship astonished – and intimidated – me. I had spent much of the previous twenty-five years engrossed in books: reading them, writing about them, writing one. My sense of self and identity had been deeply invested in academic achievement and my job as a journalist. By some unclear process of drift and a sense of inevitability, I had become a mother, and I had only the haziest idea of what that would entail. The only certain thing was that the career would continue. When a newspaper story broke a few days after the birth on a subject I knew, I put the cot at my feet and logged on to my computer. A gentle and endlessly obliging baby, Eleanor lay there while I worked all day writing the story. She didn't even get fed, I confessed anxiously to the midwife later; she seemed sleepy, so I let her be.

I appreciate now the significance of those early months. It was one of those points when life is profoundly and permanently wrenched on to a new course. At the time I was as intent on my

career as my then-husband; it was just that I (and it was predominantly me) now had this baby to fit into the demands of a
working life. But that first night in the hospital with my daughter
was the beginning of a relationship which could not be calculated in terms of cost and benefit; this was an unconditional,
open-ended commitment. This really was 'till death do us part'.

It is from our mothers and fathers that most of us first accumu-
late our embodied knowledge – the touch, feel and taste – of
being cared for. That foundational knowledge is reflected in subsequent relationships through life. The psychoanalyst Wendy
Hollway suggests care 'creates the floor of everyone's self . . . the
warp on which individuality is woven'. She maintains that 'the
care relationship is held in our bodily memories, known there
as a resource for all future encounters'.

This care relationship – parenting – is usually associated with
fulfilment and pleasure, and still commands some cultural prestige. It is a good starting point for defining care. In her work on
the philosophy of the care ethic, Virginia Held suggests that care
is not exclusive to biological mothers or to women, but is a set
of habits that help to nurture and sustain the lives of others, and
she urges that 'mothering' be a metaphor appropriate to either
sex. The philosopher of care Maurice Hamington uses an anecdote of washing his young daughter's hair. He describes how, as
he poured the warm water and lathered the shampoo, he and
his daughter told each other stories, joked and sang; 'she would
know the care and love in her body. We can communicate care
through touch, and we can remember care in a muscle memory.'
Care is 'embodied as a form of ethics which we understand
through our bodies in ways which we can't always articulate. We
start learning of care through the body as babies before we have
language.' Hamington suggests 'we are built for care'; our bodies'
physiology – senses, muscle memory, subtlety of touch, facial

expressions, ability to focus attention, sympathetic neurology – facilitate our ability to care.

Care is a form of enquiry or knowledge work, he continues, because you cannot care for what you don't know about. That also entails an ethical dimension in which you choose to know or not know for fear of the demands it might make on you. A professor of nursing education assesses applicants by their willingness to look up on a crowded train to see if someone needs their seat: there has to be a willingness to recognize need. Iris Murdoch writes that the most basic requirement for a person to be good is that they must 'know certain things about their surroundings, most obviously, the existence of other people and their claims'.

'Care is a politically embodied performance,' adds Hamington; 'every iteration has the potential to contribute to our dynamic sense of moral identity and adds to our disruptive knowledge because it pulls us out of routine and demands attention and action'. We need to know *how* to care, and that requires 'habits and capacity for inquiry': this is the starting point for competence, an essential characteristic of care. The knowledge develops by a process of action, observation and reflection. Care done well is always a creative act, incorporating innovation, adaptation and spontaneity. Washing his daughter's hair leaves him with the 'powerful thought that with every caring touch, I can enable the possibility for the replication of care'.

At home with my newborn I learnt that she did not understand her own body – burps and farts convulsed her in pain and shock – and needed me to understand and introduce her to herself. She seemed half-alien, waving her fingers like a strange sea creature wafting in water – which she had been, until a few weeks previously. We were as bewildered as each other: how do you take a baby to the toilet with you? Or manage to have a bath without having to leap out, half slathered in soap, dripping bathwater all over baby and floor, and sitting shivering and wet to breastfeed?

A path lay ahead which would teach me how to be a mother. I discovered a template buried in memories of being mothered myself, and I drew on it, consciously imitating the habits and patterns of my own mother, gradually incorporating my own understanding of care. I know now there is no end to this path, only occasional lay-bys. Every stage throws up new challenges and poses the question yet again: what is it to parent a child? How do you nurture growth and development? One moment I was hustling them out of the door to school, the next I was a pit stop as they came in late from work or disappeared to study and travel, resting for a moment to discuss a problem or stopping for a meal. I am happy that they are adventurous and independent; parenting requires you to be optional in your adult children's lives. As one psychoanalyst succinctly sums it up: motherhood is the lifelong process of 'being there to be left'. They need me to exist as they launch themselves into the world, to provide the familiarity to anchor their explorations. It sounds dull – as it should be. The task is still in progress as I write, but my best guess is that parenting becomes a courageous form of witness to their unfolding lives.

Meanwhile gaps of time are now opening up and I have some perspective on the daunting process of parenting. In the thick of it, there was precious little opportunity to stand back; the pace was brisk, the subject too emotionally absorbing and the physical toll too demanding. Crises can still plunge me back into all-consuming care, but it is possible for the first time to take stock and consider what I have learnt and what skills I need for the next stage. What is the role of a mother in the second half, and how does one end what one has begun? Why do accounts of motherhood cover those daunting first few years and then peter out? It is as if the questions about what it is to be a mother are settled relatively swiftly, whereas they are just as challenging and complex as children become adults, even if the physical demands of washing, feeding and minding are much reduced.

Looking back at my twenty-five-years of childrearing, I am bemused by how unprepared I was, and how much of it arrived as a profound shock. That's always the case, suggests Melissa Benn in *What Should We Tell Our Daughters?*: the knowledge of motherhood is 'somehow culturally buried' and has to be 'learned and forgotten, over and over again'. The early years involved a large measure of clumsy frustration. For me, it was a complete reorientation, in which the well-being of my children became my primary concern. In the process, I had to reconfigure my identity as independent, determined and ambitious. Care, the labour of love, had caught up with me, and it was shaping my life as profoundly as it had my mother's. The total dependence of these small creatures brought an awareness of the vulnerability of others, and the non-negotiable commitment that required of me. It revealed a simple, obvious truth, namely that independence was an illusion and an odd ambition. The feminism of the 1980s had taken me up a dead end.

These realizations had to be kept secret as I went back to work, when my first baby was just under four months old, as was common in the 1990s. Working mothers were too grateful for their opportunity to continue a career, too nervous of the provisional concessions to maternity leave (part-time working was frowned on), and too anxious to make demands, or even to make our mothering explicit. We self-edited, tucking our home lives neatly away during working hours, determined to show our ongoing competence and dedication. Melissa Benn suggests in *Madonna and Child* that by the 1980s and 1990s, feminists 'were schooled in toughness, the work ethic has seeped too far, too deep into our thinking'.

After the birth of my second child, the nagging sense of straddling two worlds caught up with me. It felt precarious and uncomfortable, requiring difficult conversations with bosses and childminders about hours and pay, accompanied by an anxious internal monologue about whether I was doing enough, either at home or at work. Even more difficult was the growing awareness that these worlds of job and home were profoundly at odds, and required diametrically opposed versions of me. At work, I was expected to be driven, goal-oriented and productive. I had a job that prides itself on a lack of patience. 'Make it first, make it fast,' as one newsroom slogan put it. That work culture was a more pronounced version of a culture-wide impatience, in which anything that requires waiting is viewed with a particular form of horror. But the most important thing I needed as a mother was patience, and I was desperately short of it. I had no idea how I could begin to match the patience of a close friend, whose gentle, easy-going manner with her children was a source of amazement and admiration. Having developed a character full of focus, determination and energy, I knew a lot about frustration.

The problem was time – how one used, spent and passed it. With children, events unfolded and I needed to be willing to drop or change plans. Spontaneity was important, playfulness appreciated. Not only did I find the slowness of mothering infuriating, the switching back and forth required in every working day was near impossible. I had a sense of guilty relief on those occasions when I missed bath time and came home to a quiet house. As Mrs Ramsey found in *To the Lighthouse*, 'it was a relief when they went to bed. For now she need not think about anybody. She could be herself, by herself. And that was what now she often felt the need of – to think; well, not even to think. To be silent; to be alone.'

The worst occasions were when I took work habits home; if I turned my efficient, organized self on the children, it ended in tears – mine or theirs, and sometimes all three. If there was a pile of laundry, an untidy kitchen and we needed shopping, I wanted to get it all done. Baby on hip, toddler in tow, I would rush around the supermarket, distraught at the unforeseen, such as a lost dummy, or a wailing baby. Nipping out to the shops for a pint of milk was impossible; it entailed dressing up two reluctant children in coats and shoes, and getting them to walk in a straight line. If there was a puddle to stamp in, a leaf to pull or a bright flower to stare at, the whole operation could take up to an hour.

Painfully, I learnt that parenting was about interruptions. It requires reserves of adaptability for when the plan to wash the floor is upended by a broken toy, a child falling over or a tantrum. The interruptions still continue intermittently (as I write, a text arrives from a child trying to revise: they need a sandwich at 12.35 – the precision is unusual), and they are often just as non-negotiable. This time round, it may be a broken heart, a panic attack, a failed exam or a lost job. Every event at least requires a parent to recognize its seriousness and why it feels like a crisis. A willingness to be interrupted is a measure of commitment.

Interruptions are subversive because they disrupt the goal-oriented use of time. When you are interrupted, the two dominant metaphors for time – *using* it and *spending* it – slip out of reach. Motherhood wrenches you out of this mindset and relegates you to what one feminist thinker calls the 'shadow of clock time'. In his essay 'Time, Work-Discipline and Industrial Capitalism', the historian E. P. Thompson describes how industrialization led to a precise awareness of time and its value. Children were educated to be punctual and to eschew that most heinous of sins, *wasting* time. A massive cultural shift from a 'task-based' sense of time in pre-industrial society was required to synchronize the work of large numbers of people and to commodify their labour in factories. Time was now money – to be consumed, marketed and put to use. But there was an exception to this cultural shift, Thompson announces airily: 'The rhythms of women's work in the home are not wholly attuned to the measurement of the clock. The mother of young children has an imperfect sense of time and attends to other human tides. She has not yet altogether moved out of the conventions of "pre-industrial society".' After this terse dismissal of women, he goes on to consider at much greater length the sense of time among the Nuer in South Sudan.

Thompson's extraordinary prejudice persists. The first questions that colleagues asked when they visited me after my second baby was whether I had got him into a routine yet. Chasing (the elusive) routine for a baby was setting oneself up to fail, I discovered repeatedly, but it was how a new mother hoped to claw herself back into clock-based time. Care puts one at odds with how a society understands and describes time, one of the most basic social conventions to orient people and co-ordinate activity, as one theorist puts it. Many carers end up in this uncomfortable place, out of kilter and disorientated by the unpredictable, repetitive process of caring. Paid care work, such as social care, faces an acute challenge: carers find themselves caught between clock-based time and task-based time. Half an hour may not be long enough to wash and dress a client with dementia.

The conflict over time is intensifying. Speed increasingly carries cultural prestige, argues John Tomlinson in *The Culture of Speed*, and is associated with 'reason, progress, order'. He argues that we are adopting a new concept of time: 'immediacy'. The expectation is that things happen 'without delay or lapse in time, done at once, instant'. In this culture of immediacy, we expect 'rapid delivery, ubiquitous availability and instant gratification of desire'. He writes of a 'closure of the gap which has historically separated now from later, here from elsewhere, desire from its satisfaction'. 'Immediacy' cultivates certain habits of mind, such as impatience, an appetite for multitasking and a restlessness which makes elusive the attentiveness and sense of presence often required in care.

Conflicts between time cultures are inherently political, argues the theorist Valerie Bryson. It was the nineteenth-century industrialists who castigated the labouring classes for their habit of 'wasting' time. Consumer capitalism assumes that the value of time is measured by material exchange: money earned and spent, products purchased. In his autobiography Bob Dylan referred to the American Civil War between the industrial north and the predominantly agricultural south as a 'battle between two kinds of time'.

For a carer, time often becomes something to struggle with; they can never indulge in the common fantasy of controlling it. Sometimes everything is happening at the same time – or needs to; at other times, nothing is happening and a day of pottering stretches out endlessly. This is true whether we are caring for the very sick, an elderly parent or a toddler; errands and small tasks swell to fill the day. As a young mother, I would catch myself wondering whether I was 'wasting time' and then, just as quickly, realize the absurdity of the notion: spending an afternoon with a child, a tub of water and old yoghurt pots, filling and emptying them, can variously be described as education, playing or 'doing nothing'. It was hard to defend the value of such time (although the child development books offered cheery reassurance) and I felt that I seemed to be always busy and to have nothing to show for it. Just keeping them fed, washed and bedded did not seem to me to stack up to an achievement. Adrienne Rich defines caring as 'attention to small chores, errands, work that others constantly undo, small children's constant needs'.

Time was not productive in the way I wanted; raising children and caring for them is not linear – it is cyclical and repetitive. How to find repetition rewarding is part art, part skill and part commitment. Our culture is fascinated with what is novel, exciting, stimulating and fast; entertainment is designed to meet these appetites and reinforces them. Repetition is acceptable only in a narrative of achievement, such as an athlete's training. Yet over the years, I gradually came to appreciate the recurrent habits of family life: the tidying, cooking, school pick-ups, sorting laundry and washing up, grounding me in a routine dedicated to the ongoing maintenance of life.

In 1969 Mierle Laderman Ukeles, then an art student in New York, drew up a manifesto for Maintenance Art, and offered a 'Proposal for an Exhibition entitled Care'. She asserted that as an artist, she decided what art was, and that her daily chores of cleaning, washing and changing nappies were Maintenance Art. Her proposal was that she would come into the art gallery and do all the work she usually did in the home: she would sweep the floor, wash the walls, dust and cook meals. She followed this up with a project working in the New York Sanitation Department for a decade as the self-appointed artist in residence. Out of that came 'Touch Sanitation', in which she recorded meeting the 8,500 employees of the New York Sanitation Department over a year. She shook hands with each of them and thanked them for keeping New York alive, gathering and documenting her conversations with them. The projects continued and in 2013 she reflected on her practice of Maintenance Art and Care in a speech to the cleaners of Brooklyn Museum: 'What I've been trying to do all these years is to take these things that have been behind the scenes, downstairs, things that no one will talk about, and pull them back into the zone of things to look at.' She told her audience that their work as cleaners was as much 'culture' as the artefacts and installations in the galleries.

Maintenance stood in opposition, she concluded, to the predominant preoccupation with achievement and novelty. Care defined as Maintenance Art accords well with Hannah Arendt's interpretation of wisdom as a loving concern for the continuity of the world.

Much of the most invisible care is invested in continuity, and in an age preoccupied with change – either eager for it or fearful of it – continuity is disregarded, despite the many ways we want or need it. Instead, prestige accumulates around *achievement*, a word which conveys completion and an end; the etymology is from the French: 'to perform', and 'to gain through effort' – activities regarded as essential projects of the individual. In contrast, maintenance is a work of shared endeavour, requiring routine and ongoing habits.

Motherhood is just one route into learning how to care. It may be a dominant paradigm in our culture, but others who do not have children find their own experiences of patience and attention by supporting another person's vulnerability. Two different friends offered me their accounts. Their stories had close parallels; they both took care jobs in their twenties after studying as a way to earn money – one in social care, the other as a healthcare assistant.

James worked night shifts in a Salvation Army care home after graduating from Cambridge. He told me his story one evening over a curry in an Indian restaurant.

'I did bed washes, cleaning people, enemas. There was a constant smell of urine and carbolic soap. Two of us looked after thirty clients. We put people to bed, checked on them overnight, and gave out basic medication. I enjoyed talking to the elderly patients – I'm curious and I like learning about people. I didn't get much training and I didn't learn much about nursing, but I learnt a lot about people. After eighteen months I took a job in home care, visiting elderly clients in their homes. I did this work for more than three years, fitting it around my other work. It was a real counterbalance to being twenty-three, going out clubbing and seeing girls. It taught me about patience – something I had never learnt over the course of my education. It could be really draining, especially dealing with people with dementia.

'It was a useful exploration in relation to class and my whole upbringing. I grew up in an environment in which I was constantly being served. I had a nanny when I was a child, someone cleaned the house and someone else did the garden. Then I was educated at Eton, a boarding school, and I was served there; even at Cambridge a bedder made my bed. School and university had infantilized me. In this job most of my clients were working class, some were very poor and many were people of colour. There was one man whose whole body would shake. He had worked as a pile driver, building motorways all his life – and the work had left lasting damage. His wife was very tired of caring for him. It was a wake-up call to other people's lives and their very different life experiences, and these people were my neighbours. I miss it.

'I was dealing with the reality of seeing how people's bodies fall to bits. Some experiences were very profound. I learnt about the giving of physical pleasure in a way which was not sexualized. I could hold a woman, care for her, wash her genitalia. I could see it brought comfort and pleasure and was completely asexual. When someone is really frail or ill, conversation can be challenging – you run out of things to talk about or they can't easily follow the conversation or make themselves clear, so the physical relationship can become very important. The physical stuff – dressing, bathing – is something to do. How you touch someone can become very powerful. Now, I care for my father and I enjoy the physical intimacy. When his carer is off duty, I step in. He never did any of the physical caring for me as a small child, and if I'd followed the script I was brought up with, I wouldn't be washing his bum.

'It takes a couple of hours to get him up. I have to sleep in the same room and sometimes I have to get up four times in the night to help him to the toilet. We're in this together. Sometimes he is very stubborn and selfish. It's not always easy. But we can giggle about things – it can often be playful and funny. It's curious how things come full circle.'

Ramiro's first job in the UK was as a hospital healthcare assistant. 'I had never done anything like that before. I had studied philosophy, but I needed a job which I could fit round studying. I got two weeks of training, which included simple tasks such as taking a temperature, bed-making, and how to help someone to move or eat.

'The work took me to an edge where a very raw aspect of life begins. When I was eighteen, my grandfather died of cancer, and I didn't want to visit him because I couldn't face that part of life. Later, I learnt about Buddhism and that helped, and after a while, I found I could deal with such things and I felt a call to be near that suffering. I had a sense that I wanted to be in contact with all aspects of human reality – even those which are difficult.

'The first three or four months on the wards were very stressful. There were so many things to do and a patient might be crying for attention. They didn't want drugs, they wanted human contact. They didn't want to be treated like a car being taken to the garage. Some people you couldn't help because you didn't have time. A man who had been a professor was very ill and in terrible pain. He kept asking if he could be moved, just a little this way, a little that way. The nurse finally came and told me to stop moving him, but it had brought him a few seconds of relief, or perhaps he benefited from the human contact. It was very sad. I had to ignore his calls.

'When there was a painful situation, there was no one to talk to about it. It felt very solitary. I was never on a ward long enough to get to know the other staff well, and I had no supervisor to talk to.

'One young patient had a nice girlfriend and lovely family. I asked him, what can I do to help? He said, "You can give me a new bowel." He was dying of bowel cancer. I felt the enormity of his suffering. I just had to open my heart to that pain and sadness.

'All human beings suffer and to be open to that suffering is to be open to all human beings. To acknowledge that brings me close to everyone – even someone who is too sick to speak. I learnt many things about what it is to be human. I wiped many bottoms and that degree of intimacy reminds you of the fragility of the human condition and its limitations. It was a journey for me to get to that recognition. I travelled from not wanting to know, to diving right into the heart of it, and then integrating it into how I see people. It is enriching to care for people with that vulnerability – and I see that fragility in everyone now, so when I meet someone, I can imagine them in twenty years' time or more, and how they will need help for basic things like washing and going to the loo. It has shifted the way I see people. I see youth and health now as transitory.'

The work had a profound impact on both James and Ramiro. Their stories mirrored each other in another respect: strikingly, each realized they had never spoken of it before. No one had ever been interested enough to ask about it.

Care is a currency which is in constant circulation. The Inuit see it as a balanced reciprocity which defines 'who shall do what for whom in return for who has done (or should have done) what for whom in order that in the future who will do what for whom'. The Scottish poet Iain Crichton Smith describes how in the crofting community in which he grew up on the Hebridean island of Lewis each person 'is held up in its buoyancy as a swimmer in water'. Marion Coutts captures this sentiment perfectly in *The Iceberg*, her memoir of the illness and death of her husband from a brain tumour. In the final pages, she describes an extraordinary moment shortly before he died, when they celebrated Christmas with their three-year-old son, Ev, in the hospice: 'What I am seeing is an exquisite artefact held aloft. In many homes Christmas is a ritual pattern of small occurrences, yet to make this one happen – the child, the cracker, the paper crown – in the only place where it might have had a chance of happening, multiple agencies have played a role. Opaque and transparent, I cannot count them because I do not know them all to count: consultants, surgeons, nurses, therapists, doctors, relatives, friends, colleagues, strangers, donors, supporters, volunteers. Tom and Ev on the bed are a rare work of culture, dazzlingly constructed.'

Care lacks a language in part because it is often accomplished without words, but it also sometimes needs to be wordless. Discretion and tact can be essential. The quality of the care may lie precisely in not being obvious to the recipient or any observer. Incidents of care are routinely dismissed as 'just a small thing'; deprecation runs through conversations on care like lettering runs through a stick of seaside rock: 'It was nothing.' Yet this dismissiveness can also be accompanied by recognition of its value: 'It meant so much.' The significance of the gesture exceeds its description. Care can be, in James Joyce's phrase, 'the most delicate and evanescent of moments', which serve as an epiphany, not necessarily leading to new knowledge, but to recognition of the importance of something already known. The timeliness and fitness of the gesture reveal a sincerity of feeling beyond the easy reach of words.

Someone recounted to me such a moment. Six years previously, her baby was stillborn and she nearly died from a haemorrhage. The care of the nurses held her through the grief and terror, and at one point, when she was delirious with pain-killers, they talked about her favourite brand of fig rolls. She woke the following morning to find a packet of the biscuits had been left beside her bed. A nurse had gone out in her break to buy them before her shift ended. This kindness from a stranger played an important part in her recovery over the subsequent years, she maintained.

In another anecdote, the mother of a sick child described how she could guess the quality of care each nurse would offer from the way they entered the room and closed the door. Care can be embodied in how someone moves, she said. In a noisy culture which accords great significance to talking, the wordlessness of small actions can easily be overlooked.

Care is usually regarded as menial, unimportant or too closely associated with bodily processes to be worthy of description in literature. Writers have a history of active hostility. Cyril Connolly's comment has become famous: 'There is no more sombre enemy of good art than the pram in the hall.' Jane Austen would have known as much about care as she did about marriage, given that unmarried women such as herself were the first to be called on to care for the elderly, and to nurse the sick and dying. But, unlike the question of marriage, little of the subject appears in her novels. For example, early in *Pride and Prejudice*, Jane Bennet falls ill with a fever in Mr Bingley's house. Her sister Elizabeth makes great efforts to visit and takes up the role of caring for her. The delighted reunion of the girls is described, as are Jane's symptoms, and the paragraph ends with, 'Elizabeth silently attended her.' We hear nothing of what that entailed.

In her essay *On Being Ill*, Virginia Woolf suggests that 'litera-ture does its best to maintain that its concern is with the mind; that the body is a sheet of plain glass through which the soul looks straight and clear'. She laments that illness never took its rightful place as the central theme of a novel alongside love or jealousy, and suggests a 'poverty of language' surrounds the issue. Much the same can be said of that essential corollary of illness: care. Instead, Woolf argues, 'People write always about the doings of the mind; the thoughts that come to it; its noble plans; how it has civilised the universe. They show it ignoring the body in the philosopher's turret; or kicking the body, like an old leather football, across leagues of snow and desert in the pursuit of conquest or discovery. Those great wars which it wages by itself, with the mind a slave to it, in the solitude of the bedroom against the assault of fever or the oncome of melancholia, are neglected. Nor is the reason far to seek. To look these things squarely in the face would need the courage of a lion tamer; a robust philosophy; a reason rooted in the bowels of the earth.'

The poverty of language on care has become acute. In a traffic jam behind a small van, I saw a slogan emblazoned on the back doors: 'Caring for property worldwide.' A few hours later, scrubbing a stain from a shirt, the stain remover promised to 'care' for my clothes. Care is being eviscerated of meaning, four letters exhausted by their ubiquity. The same word is used for everything from security to laundry. It is sprinkled over every commercial activity like hundreds and thousands on a cake. In an insecure world of anxious consumers, capitalism dresses itself up in the language of care. English is recognized as a rich language, but how is it that the same verb applies to commercial property maintenance and some of the most intimate moments of human relationship?

It is not just capitalism which has rolled its tanks all over the word; successive waves of managerial reform in public services have bequeathed a vocabulary in which care comes in 'packages' (that is, bits), recipients are known as 'service users' and managers rely on 'tools' created by service design and PowerPoint.

The role of the professional is to 'signpost' other services; at one meeting I shadowed, a manager advised staff to 'populate the document' with the 'likes and dislikes' of the 'service user' as a form of person-centred care: it amounted to getting to know someone with the help of tick boxes. The psychiatrist Norman Doidge warned that in medicine, 'our remote obfuscating language is a pathetic replacement for a vanishing, highly personal healer-patient relationship, an ancient archetype that is being buried. People can feel stripped of their dignity, autonomy and personhood on entering such "user-provider systems".' The bureaucracy of the welfare state has also injected anxiety about risk, compliance, safety and regulation. In the process, the word 'care' has become contaminated: the term 'children in care' has been changed to 'looked-after children'. In Alan Bennett's story *The Lady in the Van*, a social worker comes to visit him after a homeless lady has moved into his drive. 'I am not her carer, I hate caring,' he expostulates. The term 'carer' is a reductionist description of a relationship developed to suit bureaucratic need rather than lived experience. A mother of a child with Down's syndrome said she had finally brought herself to apply for Carer's Allowance, but she loathed her designation as 'the primary carer' and declared with exasperation, 'I'm her mother, not her carer! What does that make her father? Secondary carer?'

A property maintenance company is happy to claim it 'cares', while a mother and the hospitable Alan Bennett don't want anything to do with the word. There are good reasons to worry when words are bankrupted of meaning. Care always seems to be teetering on this precipice: what if we lose a language to describe those relationships of dependence in which one person sustains the well-being of another? In the novel *Nineteen Eighty-Four*, George Orwell suggests that ideas become unimaginable when the language which describes them is destroyed. In his dystopia, the constant editing of Newspeak eliminates certain words.

Orwell understood that this made some ideas simply impossible to talk, write or think about – because there is no language in which to do so. We need always to be alert for ideas which are being reconfigured, compromised or destroyed, he warned.

The word 'care' is in a double bind: historically invisible and unarticulated, and now colonized by bureaucratic and commercial imperatives. 'We need words to keep us human and our needs are made of words; they come to us in speech and they die for lack of expression. Without a public language to help us find our words, our needs will dry up in silence. Without the light of language we risk becoming strangers to our better selves,' writes Michael Ignatieff.

If the word 'care' is bureaucratized, we could lose sight of important dimensions of relationship. For example, the attentiveness required to care for someone who does not have the language or capability to express their need – a baby, an incapacitated patient on intensive care, a dementia sufferer. Close observation is required as well as interpretation and a practical response. Attentiveness can take the form of engrossment: a foster mother described her response to a troubled foster son: 'I'm listening with my eyes and ears, listening to what's being said and not said. It's every day, all the time.' Caring for someone who is acutely ill or in a crisis can entail such intense absorption in another that the carer's own sense of self becomes peripheral.

More commonly, the carer's attention holds a wide field of concern. Parents maintain an ongoing awareness of their child's physical, emotional and educational well-being, so that every issue – from friendships to dentists, from maths tests to football teams – is kept in mind. A frail elderly parent has a comparable range of needs requiring awareness: do you notice the step, the crack in the pavement, or the draught? Are they on the right medication? Are the hearing aids working?

Then there are occasions when care requires availability, a

quality of presence. One friend described a vivid childhood memory of his mother and how he played at her feet as she ironed. The sense of being cared for was implicit in her presence. Care is often described in terms of actions, but there are occasions when care is expressed by doing nothing. A social worker in palliative care described how she had to gauge when to withdraw, and when to say nothing. She talked to me about the holding of uncertainty and anxiety and allowing things to evolve without reaching for conclusions, outcomes and certainties. This kind of care as containment of powerful emotion can be immensely demanding.

Leo Tolstoy offers a moving account of such modesty in *The Death of Ivan Ilyich*. A powerful exception to Virginia Woolf's observation about the absence of illness in literature, Tolstoy's novella describes how a wealthy man dies of a painful disease, abandoned by his wife and family, his doctors, friends and colleagues. Only Gerasim, a peasant boy, a recent arrival in the household, is willing to care for Ivan Ilyich: 'For his excretions also special arrangements had to be made, and this was a torment to him every time – a torment from the uncleanliness, the unseemliness, and the smell, and from knowing that another person had to take part in it. But just through this most unpleasant manner, Ivan Ilyich obtained comfort.'

Tolstoy describes how Gerasim 'refrains from looking at his sick master out of consideration for his feelings', and when Ilyich apologizes for the unpleasantness, he replies, 'What's a little trouble? It's a case of illness with you, sir.' Gerasim is strong and healthy and yet deft, gentle and has a lightness of step. When the pain in Illyich's legs becomes intense, Gerasim raises them on to his shoulders to bring relief, communicating care through touch, gesture and movement. 'No one felt for him [Ivan Ilyich] because no one even wished to grasp his position. Only Gerasim recognized it.'

In his poem *Ash Wednesday*, T. S. Eliot articulates an uncomfortable paradox that we need to be taught to care but also not to care:

> *Blessèd sister, holy mother, spirit of the fountain, spirit of*
> *   the garden,*
> *Suffer us not to mock ourselves with falsehood*
> *Teach us to care and not to care*

The poem was dedicated to his mentally ill wife Vivienne, but at the time of writing, they were estranged and shortly afterwards became legally separated; she was later committed to a mental-health asylum by her brother. After her committal, Eliot did not see her again. This odd, sharp line resonates with a painful personal dilemma, one that many carers stumble across at some point, particularly in intimate relationships. Some are charged with exhaustion, anger and guilt. What are the limits to care? When care work is a job, Eliot's injuncture 'not to care' is essential: a doctor or nurse must be able to walk off the ward and return to the preoccupations and pleasures of his or her own life. Henry Marsh, the neurosurgeon, suggested in a radio interview that surgeons may need to be distant and cold with the patient as a form of protection that enables them to deal with the enormous risks inherent in brain surgery. But Eliot's words are also sinister. Not caring can become abuse. Indifference or neglect has consequences: an elderly patient may be given a glass of water but if it is just out of reach, the risk of dehydration is high. An absence of attention can tip an act of care into its opposite.

At a meeting of a group of volunteers at a hospice, I asked how they would define care. Over coffee, we laughed at anecdotes about our early parenting and went on to discuss the care of elderly parents, grandchildren, friends and sick relatives. One by one, they offered their experiences, and what emerged was a kaleidoscopic pattern of contrasting views drawn from culture, faith and personal biography.

Jackie was the first to speak: 'My parents came from Ireland and they could barely read or write, so as children we always cared for them. I have two grandsons and one is very empathic; when we are walking down the street, he will say that he wants to walk slowly for my sake. The other grandson is the opposite. Care seems to be something innate – you are born with it.'

Lucile disagreed. For her, it was something you learnt and it started in the home: 'My parents always helped people who were sick, whether they were near or far. As soon as we heard someone was sick, everyone would ask, what can we do to help? That was the Caribbean way, and that's how the village was when I was growing up. When I came here, I didn't want to ask for help, I was too proud, but I needed it.'

At this point, Grace interjected impatiently, 'The first person I care for is me. I have to care for myself in order to care for others. I was taken into the care system in Jamaica. I remember the judge saying that I was to be taken into "care and protection". His words were indelible on my heart. I suffered and I was determined to stop others going through that. When my stepfather and mother were like babes in my hand, I cared for them.'

Frank, a retired social worker, considered his words carefully as he spoke, 'Care is overlooked, it's an abstract concept. Care is about the soul, not just the practical issues. It enriches the giver as much as the recipient.' He described how, as a volunteer, he was visiting a man who had multiple sclerosis, and whose wife had left him. 'This man has such spirit and I find it so inspiring. Once, on a visit, I saw suitcases in the hall and the wife had come to stay before going to Africa. I asked how the man could put up with his wife treating him like that – coming and going as she wished without regard for him. "What does a woman want with a husband like me?" he said, laughing so much that I found myself laughing too. He could laugh about his terrible situation.'

'I ensured that my children cared for me as much as I cared for them,' added Jackie. 'They shared the chores; my son used to close the curtains so people couldn't see him ironing.'

Miriam, the coordinator of the project, giggled, as she gave a list of all those she cared for, in order of priority. Her cats came first, followed by colleagues, her volunteers, parents and her husband.

'The first people I care for are my parents – they cared for me and now in return I care for them. My wife and children come second, and then my neighbours. In my culture in Somalia, we respect the elderly,' said Hassan. 'I was brought up to see all my elders as auntie and uncle –' At this everyone around the table was voluble in agreement, drawing from their own cultural backgrounds. 'I believe you care for yourself by caring for others,' added Hassan.

There was widespread nodding, but Jackie pointed out that as a feminist she has for many decades seen care as the product of a framework of duty, power and respect. Then the conversation moved on to carelessness. Kate talked about how someone in the hospital had put wet socks on her aged dying mother's feet. She was still very upset. A vigorous discussion followed, criticizing the care provided by the NHS, a narrative of loss and nostalgia for a golden era in the past. Was it related to the decline of faith? asked one. No, countered another, look at the abuse of care perpetrated by religious institutions: that was not care.

The conversation could have gone on, but the coffee was finished and the biscuits eaten.

<h1 style="text-align:center">(ii)</h1>

<h2 style="text-align:center">empathy</h2>

empathy, noun – The power of identifying oneself mentally with (and so fully comprehending) a person or object of contemplation.

sympathy, noun – An expression of understanding and care for someone else's suffering.

The word most closely associated with care is 'empathy'. The term has proliferated into every area of public debate. More than 1,500 books with 'empathy' in the title are on sale on Amazon. Barack Obama declared that the 'Empathy Deficit' was the 'moral test of our times'. The American psychologist Brene Brown has explained the word to millions through her TED talks and books: 'Empathy requires us to do something and that is to draw upon our own emotional experience and to feel the other's pain,' she suggests. 'The best way to ease someone's suffering is to go down and feel it with them.' To be able to say, 'I know what it's like down there.' Her confident definitions are not supported by the word's curious history.

The word 'empathy' was only coined in 1909 by the psychologist Edward Bradford Titchener to translate the German word *Einfühlung*, best understood as 'feeling one's way into'. At this stage, the word was not about feeling another person's emotion, but about projecting one's imagined feelings on to the world. Early empathy experiments focused on a bodily feeling or movement that produced a sense of merging with an object. Psychologists later redefined the word to apply to relationships between people. The *Reader's Digest* used the term in 1955, defining it as the 'ability to appreciate the other person's feelings without yourself becoming so emotionally involved that your judgement is affected'. These definitions did not indicate any ethical imperative – that has been added. In recent decades, empathy has been redefined again as a physiological capability identifiable in part of the brain which, like a muscle, can be developed. The word's meaning has shifted several times in its short history, claims social psychologist C. Daniel Batson, and now applies to eight different phenomena. An article in *The Atlantic* magazine suggested, 'Ask your friends for a definition and watch the meanings proliferate.'

The concept is now used to answer two very different questions: how can someone infer what another is feeling? And what might move someone to help another who is suffering? The first is about knowledge, the second is about ethical behaviour, and one cannot assume there is a link between the two – the skill of the torturer may lie precisely in their capacity for empathy. The psychologist Theresa Wiseman researched a wide range of jobs which required empathy and concluded that it entailed four characteristics: to take the perspective of another; to stay out of judgement; to recognize the other's emotion; and to communicate that recognition. Forty years ago, competence and respect might have been deemed sufficient in a doctor or nurse, but expectations have risen, and now patients and their families want evidence of empathy.

The idea that it is possible to instruct a workforce in the display of emotion (and measure it) was first developed in business. Empathy audits are standard in many retail companies, and these ideas were imported into public services, particularly healthcare, in the 2000s. One NHS policy instructed nurses to smile more. Explaining the initiative, the health secretary said, 'One of the things which came out of the focus-group discussions was that they didn't feel nurses gave the impression that they cared enough. They felt they should smile more.' He promised that nurses' 'empathic care' would be measured and scores published online in a 'compassion index'. Several countries have developed 'empathy laboratories' in which people can take on the role of patient in simulated contexts to develop deeper understanding. The danger is that expectations of empathy prompt a form of performance – what a palliative-care doctor described as the 'well-practised head tilt'.

Perhaps these expectations of demonstrating emotion place too high a burden on medical professionals: several studies of nurses and doctors in training show a decline in empathy as they work with patients. One nurse put it eloquently when she said she felt beaten down by the definitions of care and the emotions expected to accompany it: 'I take care of people I can't stand. I don't care a hoot about them. I would prefer never to see them again, but what I do care about is doing a really good job and giving really good physical care to all my patients.' Gavin Francis, a GP and author, urges that 'if physicians are to be effective in relieving suffering, a balance needs to be found between paucity and excess of empathy'. He suggests that it should be shown 'to the right person, at the right extent at the right time.' The doctor and author Raymond Tallis points out that doctors 'are taught how to *perform* the role of a good – listening, caring, empathic – doctor. Sincerity is beside the point. The doctor has to develop a manner of empathy regardless of their feelings.' The old adage used to be that people rarely sued a doctor who smiled a lot, and the performance may influence the patient's judgement of their care more than the outcome.

*

Empathy has largely supplanted the older word 'sympathy'. Both incorporate the Greek word for suffering, *pathos*. The Enlightenment philosopher David Hume argued for the link between emotion and ethical action through sympathy: someone could feel the pain of another and thus be moved to help. 'The minds of men are mirrors to one another, not only because they reflect others' emotions, but also because those rays of passions, sentiments and opinions may be often reverberated and decay away by insensible degrees.' Our emotional lives are interlinked, and that subjectivity can become interpersonal, a shared felt experience between people. Such emotional responses are not always conducive to calm and competent care, however, as Hume acknowledges. He was so overcome with 'sympathy' when observing a surgical operation that he had to leave the room.

Virginia Woolf ridiculed the concept of sympathy, briskly announcing in her essay *On Being Ill* that 'we can do without it. That illusion of a world so shaped that it echoes every groan, of human beings so tied together by common needs and fears that a twitch at one wrist jerks another, where however strange your experience other people have had it too, where however far you travel in your own mind someone has been there before you – is all an illusion. We do not know our own souls, let alone the souls of others. Human beings do not go hand in hand the whole stretch of the way. There is a virgin forest, tangled, pathless, in each; a snow field where even the print of birds' feet is unknown. Here we go alone, and like it better so. Always to have sympathy, always to be accompanied, always to be understood would be intolerable.'

Sympathy had been tainted by its Victorian popularity and is still struggling to escape from that heritage of sentiment and condescension. Brene Brown, as a prophet of empathy, dismisses sympathy as a way of distancing, but the American philosopher

Martha Nussbaum takes a different stance, urging a revival, precisely because it takes an ethical stance. Significantly, Brown uses metaphors of electricity and fibre-optics, talking of empathy 'fuelling connection'. It's the language of intensity but also, literally, consuming, and loaded with the uncertainty about reliability characteristic of digital communications – will I get cut off? Hume and other Enlightenment thinkers used a gentler metaphor, likening how we feel another's pain to the reverberation of strings on an instrument.

3

Listening to Vivaldi

IN THE CHARITY

*'There was a television drama on autism
and I just couldn't watch it. They were using
for entertainment things which I have lost,
and which most people are not even aware of
having. It was just too painful.'*

SALLY, the mother of a son with autism

I travelled north to the offices of a voluntary-sector organization which offered support to families of children with a disability. Nothing prepared me for the intensity of the time I spent there. I was to shadow appointments, visit families in their homes and interview staff for a few days. The cramped offices tucked into a basement on a side street of a busy city came to represent an electricity substation in my mind, but instead of routing power, it was handling emotions which could capsize lives and bureaucratic procedure. Grief, anger, fear, shame, frustration: this was the raw stuff of the organization's working day. Listening was their first task, then the hard slog over months, or even years, of helping families navigate their way through complex bureaucracies of health, education and social services to fight for the care for their child. The cases that arrived at the charity's door were the toughest: children who did not fit any straightforward diagnosis, parents overwhelmed by the interactions with professionals and the needs of their child. The charity was caught at the interface between desperate families and an overstretched system of services hit by budget cuts and intent on rationing care.

Over the course of the meetings and interviews, I saw care provided in three different ways: by parents, the state services and the charity itself. Frequently there was bitter and passionate conflict between parental care and the differing perspectives of the professionals in health, education and social work; care was repeatedly likened to a battlefield. Across the country, parents comment on the adversarial nature of getting provision for their disabled child, and many resort to lawyers to fight their case.

This charity had grown out of a support group for parents with a disabled child, and sought to offer solidarity and advocacy to families who were often at breaking point; at any one time they supported up to 800 families. Above all, it was a work of witness, and it exacted a heavy toll on the charity's staff. One explained how he was routinely dealing with tragedy and injustice, and likened the emotional intensity of the job to armed conflict. I had arrived in a place of crisis, both in individual families' lives, but also in the systems set up to provide care. At the end of my visit, I was emotionally drained, overwhelmed by the task facing staff and parents in this force field of suffering, and humbled by their determination and capacity for endurance.

The majority of parents coming to the charity for support were women. Several I interviewed had been left by their partners and were raising their children alone. Some were traumatized by their struggle, but they wanted to talk, and sometimes at great length. To my surprise, all of them thanked me profusely for listening. 'It has been cathartic to talk,' said one – a sentiment echoed by others – and she added that she rarely spoke of the harrowing incidents which dominated her days and nights. 'It's another world,' as one mother put it.

This world is little understood, with few translators and even fewer visitors. It requires parents to learn a foreign language of acronyms, medical terms and bureaucratic procedures. Fights over diagnoses, respite care, equipment and educational provision can last years.

These mothers talked of lost friendships, relatives who withdrew, and many of the normal activities of family life beyond reach. The parents learn to edit their lives; the suffering is too intense and unfamiliar for many relatives, friends and colleagues to bear. When their child did not meet developmental 'milestones', they found themselves cut off and isolated. Visits to a restaurant, playground or cinema were an ordeal; strangers misjudged, tutted and disapproved, uncomprehending. The parent becomes a buffer zone to protect the child – the mediator, the translator and the defender. The prodigious effort can go unrecognized by anyone. They have to dig deep into inner resources to find meaning for their struggle. In *Love's Labor*, the American feminist philosopher Eve Feder Kittay writes about her disabled daughter, Sesha, and asks for a redefining of normality that accepts her unique individuality but accepts that 'at the same time I have to see the child as others see her so that I can mediate between her and the others to negotiate acceptability. The parental task involves then socializing the child for acceptance, such as it might be, of the world, and socializing the world, as best you can, so that it can accept your child.'

A painful aspect of many stories was the family's loss of privacy. Raising a disabled child opens up the most private aspects of family relationships to professional scrutiny, analysis and judgement. A basic element of parenting – that the parent is the best authority on their child – is challenged. The professionals' personal prejudices can spill into judgement across a broad front; I was told that parents had been held to account for their choice of where to live, how to look after their house, their style of parenting and their eating habits. Add in differences of class and literacy, and the sense of humiliation can be profound and lasting.

One of the most basic assumptions of having a new baby is that the child will be a source of pleasure. 'Enjoy!' the midwife said to me as I left hospital. It jarred at the time because it echoed consumer service, as if this baby was a meal being brought to my table. But what if the parents of the newborn are dealing with grief, not pleasure? How does this change the relationship of care? As I listened to these mothers, I glimpsed how they had found their own ways to define care. Alongside their determination and endurance, they celebrated whenever the circumstances allowed, and enjoyed the normal wherever it was possible. Failures of many kinds were unavoidable, I was told, a frequent part of daily life. 'There are no happy endings,' one mother made a point of emphasizing – often there is not even an ending in sight. The struggle can last a lifetime, with no miraculous cures, just a day-to-day persistence to maintain dignity and meaning.

Sam enjoyed her career in the book trade and delayed having a child until her mid-thirties. Having a child with Down's syndrome turned her life upside down.

'After he was born, I grieved very intensely for the challenges he would face. His father coped differently. He would make hurtful remarks about our son, such as not liking his expression. I spent that first year trying to defend our son from his father's criticisms. He was in mourning and then, after that year, he accepted the diagnosis. He loves his son dearly.

'From the time he was two, I knew he wasn't like other Down's children, and at first I thought it was my fault. It was me, it was my mothering. I had never wanted to be a mother – my then-husband had wanted children – and I questioned my own ability. His first year at mainstream primary school was intolerable. He was overwhelmed by the scale of the place, the number of children, and the noise. It was a multisensory overload. I found it difficult to explain my concerns. You are met with sighs – another fussy, middle-class mum. I found the labelling very difficult. I worked very hard at trying to be clear, and to understand where the professionals were coming from. I kept thinking that if I, a professional, educated woman, found it difficult, then how much worse must it be for others.

'It falls more heavily on the mothers – they do the heavy lifting, such as dealing with the bureaucracy. Getting the autism diagnosis when he was six was late, but it was a relief – it meant it wasn't my mothering. Now I had strategies to use, and I could choose my battles. A dual diagnosis is very helpful: no one argued with us about special provision.

'We talk of "chronic sorrow" of parents with a child with additional support needs. It can easily be triggered. I had six years of grief before I began to reach adjustment. I'm in a period of grief now, because he is coming up to the end of school. I love celebrating things with him – birthdays, for example. My son loves dancing, so when he was in a show, I brought flowers and photographed him on the doorstep. He loves that.

'You don't know how your child will be received in the world. There is no guarantee of a welcome for my child. I'm often pleasantly surprised by young people in coffee shops, who are friendly and relaxed. You have to listen very closely to my son when he speaks, and he can be quite random. He is amusing,

and that's endearing to people, but with autism, he has no interest in other people. When he was younger, I felt I was translator
and interpreter between him and the world.

'At times I struggled to shift the sense of shame. I was
ashamed that I was grieving for a child who was alive and right in
front of me. I was fearful for his future and I was not celebrating
him. I needed to have a place where I could talk about my son
and encounter no judgement, just compassion, and that's why I
ended up working at this charity for a while. I was surrounded
by other mothers in a similar situation and we all supported each
other. At times, we were all weeping, but it was an incredibly
affirming environment. I changed my work and trained as a
counsellor for parents with disabled children. I've worked with
parents whose great fear is that their child is not lovable. I've sat
with them in their profound grief that their child is not loved in
the world – that's corrosive to the soul.

'There is a huge amount of scrutiny; you lose the privacy of
your parenting and family life. People come into your home a lot
and they look at how tidy it is or how nice. I knew mums who
ran around to get their homes clean before the physiotherapist
arrived. They wanted to look like they were coping – it was part
of their self-respect – that they could hold things together as a
mother.

'Amongst working-class mothers, I think there is a lot of fear
that their children might be taken away. Judgements about class
are evident; in one case I witnessed, there were clearly issues
in the family, but the social workers seemed overawed and dis-
tracted by the beautiful, comfortable house. In the end, it's a
lottery with the professionals. Some doctors, social workers and
teachers are compassionate, others not.

'Having difficult or negative emotions about our children is
really uncomfortable, but if we don't express them, they leak
into our behaviour. The big issue about autism is that it feels

personal; for example, if he's lying down in the street, there's a tendency to think, why is he doing this to me? I had to put a light on the difficult feelings provoked by comparing my life, my child, my options. I had to do some reframing. Shame loves the darkness, loves secrets. You have to let the light in and talk.

'The process is one of first acknowledging, then adjusting and adapting, and you have to do that at every life stage of your child. It's an isolated process, because your child is not meeting social expectations. You might have to acknowledge: this is not what I wanted. That can sometimes feel like a betrayal of my child.

'It has been a journey of great complexity and depth. What I have come to realize is that we are all interdependent, yet dependency is stigmatized. I want this story out there; it's part of the human experience, so it belongs to us all.'

Kate is a gentle, soft-spoken woman. She works for the charity and also has a child with additional needs. She smiles with a kind of brave cheerfulness, but the sadness is palpable.

'My son seemed normal when he was born. It crept up on us that he wasn't developing; the diagnosis of autism is so vague and we didn't get one until he was four.

'Caring for autism is emotionally wearing; my son is now fifteen and has very low levels of empathy. He can do something aggressive and is not aware of its emotional impact. It's hard to explain to other people this lack of reciprocity. If I'm ill or have hurt my back and we can't go out, he'll get so angry he will rip the curtains down.

'Another family might have been more organized and calmer. You can only be yourself. At least we have been very proactive, finding solutions, teaching him to talk. We have spent a lot of time and money trying to teach him; sometimes it went well, sometimes it just seemed to annoy him.

'The house used to get smashed up every week, and it's

been flooded. We've had to get multiple sets of new curtains and carpets, five new televisions. Innumerable lamps have been smashed. That's all on top of us getting hurt as well. It's been much worse since he became a teenager. On occasion, we have had to turn the power off, switch the water off, even let him smash up a chest of drawers. One time he took a bed apart. It's unpredictable. Things can go all right for a month or two, and then it's bad for a week. The triggers can be tiny – it is raining, or someone comes up to him too quickly, or a barking dog.

'We were snowed in once, and my son couldn't cope. It took three months to get him to calm down. You can distract small children, but as he's got older his anxiety has got worse. We can only do a narrow range of things. Sometimes we go on holiday or to a concert and within fifteen minutes we realize it's not going to work.

'There is often a lack of acknowledgement of the emotional trauma of bringing up someone who lacks empathy and has difficult behaviour. The professionals don't seem to understand: we've gone to people, quite desperate, and we've been told that we already get more services than others – but maybe we need them. We finally had to admit that we couldn't look after him. It needs a team of people who aren't exhausted. He is at a residential school now and there are a lot of staff. It has been wonderful for him. For the first time we are getting some relief. A few months ago, we had our first week off in fifteen years, because he is now a weekly boarder.

'My son likes cycling, riding, cooking, cleaning, he can dress himself, but he's not good at the academic side of things. We love the things he can do – he's very tall and looks very healthy and fit. He loves the outdoors.

'People try to give you a happy ending, but I'm still frazzled and tired. It's hard to have so much invested in someone who seems so uninterested in you. I think my husband and I are quite fragile. We feel traumatized. We are prone to anxiety and my husband has a diagnosis for mild post-traumatic stress disorder. Sometimes I can't sleep and I wake up screaming, clutching things. We've had years when we don't know if he will go to sleep and when. There were times in the past when we might have got three good nights' sleep a month. People used to ask what we do when we have respite care, and my answer was really simple: things like sleep or going for a walk.

'Even now, week in and week out, we live in a very unstable situation. My son is due back from school for four days. It could be lovely, or we could be holding the door shut to protect ourselves while he smashes the room up.

'There can be times when it's funny. We took him to the park recently and he kept repeating, "Boy wants Coca-Cola." He must have said it 300 times, but when we got to the café, he asked for a Fanta. My husband and I fell about laughing. We've developed an appreciation of his quirks – they can be funny. There are loads of things we really love about him, but we have these really terrible incidents. Quite a lot of people meet him and think he is a charming child, but then they haven't been dragged across the room by their hair. We've all been changed by it. My daughter has had to support us a lot. We will be working through this for the rest of our days.

'We don't socialize much anymore – people don't come over. That spontaneity has drained out of our lives. I could have done so much more for my mother when she was elderly, but I was always fighting on the home front. My brother doesn't get involved, but my husband's two brothers have been supportive; at least they still invite us all over. My sister said, "You are welcome, but don't bring your son."

'The interactions with the Department of Work and Pensions are like running a small business. I estimate it takes about a day a week. It's difficult enough for me, but what about someone who has problems with reading and writing? You're fighting all the time as they attempt to make cuts. You have to do the application for the Disability Living Allowance every few years. When you call the DWP, you end up listening to Vivaldi for twenty minutes.

'The DLA form is fifty-odd pages, and it looks like a small telephone directory. The first time I couldn't fill it in on my own, it was so depressing. I was in deep grief at his diagnosis – if I'd known how much worse it was going to get, I'd have been heartbroken. A social worker took pity on me and helped. You have to summarize what is your child's worst day. You have to recount every horrific aspect of your child's disability on the form. The families' tendency is to understate, because that is how they cope.

'I've worked in this world for a long time and I've seen a constant chipping away in services from both the state and the voluntary sector over the last twenty-five years. Most social workers are sympathetic, but they have less to offer and feel powerless and they tend to push it back on to the family. You get offered too much advice and too little support.

'At the moment, we're fighting a running battle because when a child goes into residential care, your benefits go into chaos, and you have to reapply for some benefits such as the Carer's Allowance. I now have to fill out a form every six weeks to account for the days he was home, and then they recalculate the benefits. Once they forgot to pay and my Carer's Allowance took months to sort out – so it was back to Vivaldi for five months.

'We've had a battle with the psychiatrists and psychologists about his medication as well. We wanted to see if the school could help him before they started using medication; we wanted as few drugs as possible. We held the line.

'Christmas and New Year is a nightmare. There is no respite on offer and no play schemes are running. It feels like everyone is having a good time except for you. People invite you to their parties, but they would be devastated if you turned up with your child. I would be so anxious that my child would do something inappropriate anyway. We socialize with other families with children with a severe disability because you all understand what you are coping with.

'Both my husband and I are very strong-willed. I think others might have given up on aspects of our son's life, but we have given him the best life we can. We have both thrown our own lives under the bus in the process. I wouldn't wish what we've been through on my worst enemy.'

The following day I bumped into Kate again, and she had drawn me a map of the different professionals and institutions she dealt with. The page of A4 was covered with neat labels and arrows. It was like the organogram of a small organization, and one of its main departments seemed to be a public relations agency. Kate said she and her husband made a point of trying to develop cordial relationships with the professionals assigned to their case, and had succeeded, with one exception when they insisted an incompetent social worker was taken off their case.

The interface is often fraught with potential conflict between the family and the professionals and bureaucrats who run services. On the one hand, there are the intense private emotions of individuals, and on the other, forms of professionalism designed to be objective, and follow procedure. Services for children with special needs are structured in silos of health, education and social services and, despite repeated attempts to improve co-ordination, the families sometimes find themselves battling on several fronts, with a frequently changing cast of professionals. Often the parents come to be seen as a problem by the professionals, rather than the child's most dogged advocates, a point made by a savagely critical report in 2019 by the parliamentary

Joint Committee on Human Rights. It described the 'horrific reality' of conditions and treatment in mental-health hospitals for young people with learning disabilities and autism, with frequent use of physical restraint and solitary confinement. The inadequacy of community-based care led to inappropriate detention which 'inflicted terrible suffering on those detained, causing anguish to their distraught families'. The report also criticised an ineffectual inspection system, which left it to the media and parents to expose the cruelty.

It can be easier if there is a clear biomedical diagnosis. One of the charity's clients, a mother of a haemophiliac child, described close collaboration with medical staff, which contrasted sharply with the accounts of the mothers of children with developmental disabilities. But she emphasized how she had worked hard to maintain the relationship, giving the professionals the benefit of the doubt when treatment was clumsy or mistakes were made. She knew it had worked because the hospital commented on the notes that her family was 'tolerant'. When there is no clear diagnosis, the scene can be set for a long and bitter struggle. One mother of a son with autism told me it had been 'ten years of being told off and told what to do'.

Much of the charity's caseload consisted of the casualties of underfunded care systems. Local-authority social-work departments and social-care budgets have had to deal with a succession of cuts under austerity; as early as 2012, the British Association of Social Workers warned that unmanageable caseloads were posing an 'imminent and serious risk to the people who need services', and more than half of social workers feared that lack of support could have tragic consequences for service users. Unlike many other areas of public services, such as education and health, social-work budgets did not benefit from the Labour government spending in the 2000s, and yet they were hard hit, along with other areas of local-authority expenditure, under austerity. Across the country, services and jobs were cut. The number of nurses trained in learning disabilities dropped by 40 per cent between 2010 and 2018, and new applicants have also fallen as the jobs disappear. By 2017, a survey of social workers painted a dramatic picture of how they had been expected to implement cuts, with nearly 70 per cent reporting that managers wanted them to ration care. A third acknowledged that they couldn't get people the care they needed, and a quarter were unsure that the care packages were even 'fair and safe'. The report noted that the 'system was buckling' and that 'it was clear that in some places the law is being at best "bent", at worst systematically breached, as local authorities scrabble to fulfil their legal duties with grossly insufficient resources.' It warned that 'officials were coming up with ever more creative and sometimes frankly absurd ways of restricting the ways in which precious social-care funding can be spent'.

In 2014 a new law, the Children and Families Act, brought hope. After listening to parents of disabled children, the government promised to meet their requests for earlier support and a less adversarial system; the new code of practice said that needs would be 'picked up at the earliest point with support routinely put in place quickly'. The high hopes quickly faded as local authorities struggled to find the funds to implement their new statutory duties. Three quarters of parents said they had found it hard to get educational support, and many had had to hire lawyers to help them, research found in 2016. The average wait for a diagnosis of autism was three and half years. Parents resorted to fighting all the way to the Special Educational Needs and Disability (SEND) tribunal, where cases were repeatedly found in favour of parents. In a notorious incident in 2016, Baker Small, a law firm which had contracts with several local authorities, including Buckinghamshire, Norfolk and Gloucestershire, tweeted gloatingly of victories over parents in SEND tribunal cases; its insensitivity attracted national media coverage, which pointed out that the company's website boasted of helping councils cut costs. Parents had long complained of the company's adversarial style.

By late 2018, it was reported that councils were having to raid other educational budgets, such as early-years funding, to plug a gap in funding for SEND. Southwark council said, 'Funding from central government doesn't come close to paying for the support that is needed.' Some councils cut budgets, and then found themselves facing legal challenges from parents, after a successful legal action in Bristol over a £5 million cut in 2018. One tragic outcome was that children with SEND were disproportionately likely to be excluded or illegally 'off-rolled' (when parents are asked informally to remove their child from school); cuts in support staff meant that early intervention was not in place to prevent challenging behaviour escalating to the point of exclusion. Boys with SEND were nearly four times more likely than other pupils to be permanently excluded.

A disturbing picture emerged of a laudable legislative ambition which lacked the necessary funding, leaving local authorities with new responsibilities but without the means to fulfil them. The lobbying of politicians and voluntary-sector organizations is focused on passing the legislation, whereas its implementation in dozens of local authorities attracts much less attention. The result is a strange disconnect between the ambition of lawmakers and the reality encountered on the ground. This is exacerbated by the painful irony that research in the last thirty years has established a better understanding of many disabilities such as autism, and of effective forms of intervention, education and development. Families have been caught in the painful gap between what is now known to be beneficial and what is available.

Part of the social worker's job has always been to ration care, but when budgets shrink, this aspect of the work dominates. Gatekeeping, managing the queue, and referrals to other services can take up to 80 per cent of resources, according to some research. Cuts left social workers with large caseloads and reduced administrative staff, and the struggle to record every interaction with clients on computer systems that crash or freeze, leaving little time for building relationships. One social worker I interviewed described the traumatic process of having to cut support on which desperate families depended. Having been trained to provide care, he was leading a team of social workers who were charged with finding ways to provide its opposite – *carelessness*. The contradictions were so painfully acute he had a breakdown, and finally left social work and retrained in another field. His case was not unusual: 40 per cent of social workers (75 per cent are women) told researchers they were planning to leave the profession; the turnover rate in many teams can be a third annually.

Austerity policies have stripped a system to its bones, starving it of the essential time needed to build strong relationships. This underinvestment in relationships is a pervasive characteristic of the welfare state. Again and again, parents described professionals as judgemental, tactless and insensitive, and the impersonal nature of services as callous, even cruel. Bureaucracies are built around managing risk, impartiality, accountability and budget restraint. They follow procedures to standardize decision-making with the aim of fairness. That makes them cumbersome and unresponsive to individual needs. One of the primary tasks of the professionals encountering families with a disabled child is to assess need, and they do so using bureaucratic procedures. For the Disability Living Allowance mentioned by Kate, information provided by the parent is translated into a score.

Many of the parents I interviewed mentioned their horror of this form, and how it forced them to think of their child in ways

which they were profoundly reluctant to do, as it reduces the
child to their disabilities and resulting need. One of the main
tasks of the charity's staff is to offer help filling in the form's
dozens of pages. According to Kate, the process is inherently
demeaning and depersonalizing: 'Bureaucracies operate to crush
people who don't fit in, even those who are confident professionals. We have had a senior hospital consultant in tears, and,
on another occasion, an A & E consultant couldn't fill in the
Disability Living Allowance form – it was too distressing. They
had an emotional block over having to present their child as a
failure, stating all the things the child could not do. What parent
is prepared to do that? I've never been to a DLA meeting with
a parent without them ending up in tears. Parents are always
trying to defend their child against the diagnosis. The latter is
reductive; it can't convey what you know of the child's lovability
and recognizable humanity.'

Even amongst the original architects of the welfare state, there
was concern that state bureaucracies might ill serve the unpredictable and messy reality of the human need for care. As Sidney
Webb admitted, 'State services are apt to be blunt and obtuse, to
have no fingers, only thumbs'. William Beveridge, who drew up
the great reports which became the blueprint of the welfare state
under the 1945 Labour government, grew increasingly alarmed
as his bold reforms were implemented: 'It did frankly send a
chill to my heart,' he said on hearing that all services would be
administered by civil servants. He had hoped that friendly societies, the great invention of Victorian industrialization, would
play a role. Colleagues, anxious to ensure complete impartiality,
overruled him, and the postwar Labour government used the
wartime model of big centralized bureaucracies to run the new
services of the welfare state. A concerned Beveridge published
a much-neglected report in 1946 urging that the new structures

should not overlook the power of citizens and communities, and argued that distant, hierarchical institutions were not best placed to assess need or find solutions. Picking up Beveridge's argument in 2018, social reformer Hilary Cottam suggested that this had been the 'fatal flaw' in Beveridge's much-lauded plans for the welfare state. Too late, he 'realized he had designed people and relationships out of the welfare state', she suggests in *Radical Help*; 'they were thought at best not to matter, and at worst to be a hindrance to social progress'. The political philosopher Hannah Arendt echoed Beveridge's concern, and warned that twentieth-century bureaucracies have a form of 'mindlessness' built in, because they operate mechanically, according to rules and regulations. In such a system, 'technical expertise gets prioritized over human values', suggests political scientist David Runciman, who adds that 'the great danger of modern democracy is that it gets detached from meaningful human input and it acquires an artificial life of its own. Human beings still make the key decisions, but they do so without creative insight.'

A moving exhibition in 2019 on the history of care in the London borough of Brent over the last 150 years underlined the significance of Beveridge's regret. Some of the earliest exhibits told the story of the Foresters, a friendly society found in many towns around England. Amongst the society's embroidered sashes, banners and ceremonial axes were an ivory gavel, brown and worn with use, and a battered ledger. Debate and accountability underpinned the principles of mutuality, and were central to the collective provision of care. Friendly societies were an early form of insurance; members made small contributions to ensure provision for them and their families when they were sick or died. Branches proliferated in nineteenth-century Britain in what were known as 'courts', groups of members who lived within two miles, making it easy to collect dues and to distribute resources swiftly. Drinking rituals ensured that many members knew each other, strengthening the commitment to reciprocity. What impressed Beveridge was how the friendly societies spread rapidly in urban industrial Britain; by 1913, 75 per cent of the British workforce belonged to a friendly society, more than to the trade unions and the Methodist church combined. They were one of the most powerful and flexible working-class institutions. In place of the old rural parish system of welfare, friendly societies invented a new form of reciprocity and belonging which was effective amongst urban, mobile populations.

In 1945, in the aftermath of victory in the war, faith in central planning and the bureaucratic state was at an all-time high, and local, small, relational organizations were swept aside as a swathe of friendly societies and charities were amalgamated into state services. What emerged were patronizing and authoritarian top-down professional hierarchies. Since the 1980s, reform initiatives to overcome the shortcomings of bureaucracy have encouraged public services to mimic consumer businesses; services are expected to perform much like a commercial service. New styles of management were brought in to tighten central control and improve efficiency. The result was an increasingly transactional culture, further strangling the chance of developing the strong relationships which Cottam argues are essential to tackling many challenges now facing care in Britain. She advocates a radical redesign of welfare so that relationship is central and the recipient of services is empowered to make the key decisions over their care – recruiting the professionals themselves and developing with them the support needed.

The charity I was observing has evolved to fill the gaps in the existing state provision. Above all, they offered a relationship; they listened to the parents. At times, the help was practical, and they offered advice and served as advocates in complex cases, but often they offered solidarity in an heroic struggle. Many of the staff had first-hand experience of living with disabled children, and instead of the indifference or hostility parents commonly experienced in public, they did not judge, but offered acceptance and encouragement.

I shadowed one of the charity staff on a visit to Kim, in her home on an estate on the city outskirts. On our arrival, she plunged into an account of a series of crises involving interactions with the police and social and educational services. Slowly the story took shape. Her teenage son had, at different times, attacked his grandmother, a little cousin, a sister, an educational psychologist, and some neighbours. Kim had had health problems of her own, and had another child with a disability. She admitted to allowing mail to pile up unopened, as she was too fearful of getting information relating to her own history of cancer. She broke down in tears as she recounted her fear that she might get sent to prison because she had got in a muddle over her benefits. An intelligent and capable woman had been overwhelmed by the practical and emotional complexity of caring for her children.

The focal point of attention in the sitting room, as her daughters and her mother came and went during our long interview, was a new baby, Kim's granddaughter. She was dressed in a beautiful pink knitted cardigan. Baby paraphernalia lay around us. Four generations of women in the family hovered over the baby; motherhood was central to their identities. Above Kim's head were large photographic portraits in gilt frames of her three children as smiling toddlers.

As Kim recounted trauma after trauma – at times with flashes of bitter humour – the narrative structure was that of a spiral, as she circled round, repeating stories, adding new detail. Her son was in a residential home two and half hours away, and on heavy medication. Kim worried about the use of restraint and seclusion to manage his behaviour. He was likely to continue into adult psychiatric care, and a lifetime of institutional care. Kim was distraught at the loss: 'The bond is going. I love him, but I don't have the confidence to deal with him. I'm even starting not to miss him.'

She broke down and left the room to regain composure, but when she returned, she was still crying. 'Other people make decisions for him, such as whether he needs shoes, or his hair cutting. It strips you of being his parent. After a good visit, I still ask myself why he can't come home. I know it's not possible, because there are too many people at risk here.'

When the interview came to an end and I got up to leave, Kim said, 'Thank you for listening. I like talking about him.' It was the last part of mothering she had left. As we drove back into the city, I passed a sign in large neon letters: EVERYTHING WILL BE ALL RIGHT. It glowed in the grey rain of late afternoon.

Liz was full of humour and had a quick, pretty smile. She worked as a graphic designer and we met over lunch. She ate little, as she was so consumed with recounting her story. Despite her ready laughter, the account was wretched. On the day we met, she declared herself ecstatic: she had finally won the right of appeal on the provision of her son's education. She felt it was acknowledgement of something she knew many years ago: 'He wasn't right early on – he used to keep swiping at my cup of tea and his tantrums were spectacular; he would bang his head against the wall. When I contacted the GP and the health visitor, they said I was a first-time mum and that I worked full time. They said I was stressed and suggested I cut down on my hours. I cried with rage on the telephone.

'Finally, when he was three, I got a referral to the paediatrician, but she told me not to be silly. He is not a classic case of autism. When he was four and a half, we finally got a diagnosis that he was on the autism spectrum and I sobbed with relief. I had an explanation. He looks normal, and he appears very plausible, so his diagnosis has been questioned repeatedly. He has had nineteen reports from four paediatricians over the years, but no one has come to any clearer conclusion about the diagnosis.

'As he grew up, he would recite whole scenes from *Star Trek*. If I took him to the park, he would scream and terrorize the other children. But I was told to let him go to a mainstream school. I was naive and did what they suggested. I didn't know any better. It's the biggest regret I have. He has been trapped ever since.

'People use the word "mild" in his diagnosis, but he is really challenging. He has poor concentration. Other parents complain about how he gets obsessive about their children. His language has been very colourful, much to my embarrassment. Parents used to say to me, "Your child needs a good slap." That really bothered me, I was being judged.

'One day there was a meltdown in the playground because the school shirt I had bought didn't have a logo. He was shouting and screaming and the other mothers stood and watched. They had no idea what it was like to be in my shoes.

'He was treated in his school like a badly behaved boy rather than someone with autism. The meetings with the school were awful; you could feel the hostility the minute you walked into the room. The learning assistant said that my son "just couldn't be bothered, couldn't be motivated"; they didn't know the basics of how to deal with autism. Eventually the paediatrician told the school he had Asperger's, and dyspraxia as well.

'He sees himself as normal; he is always trying to be like his peers and conceal his disability. We battled to get people to accept his problems and there were things we missed. He would come home and vent his frustration. He was nine years old and sobbing his heart out. Once, I even found him with a belt around his neck. He kept saying he didn't want to live. He was diagnosed as having a severe depressive disorder and they put him on medication.

'He is now in his third year of secondary school and things have gone really wrong. I'm so angry. Inclusion hasn't worked; the teachers just revert to their usual way of working. He finds things like assembly really difficult, because there's too much noise. He's a large lad now, over six foot. Several members of staff say they feel threatened, and he has been excluded several times. At one meeting, the headteacher finally agreed with us, and was honest enough to say we'd been failed.

'He can be violent. He pinned me up against the wall once when I took his mobile away. I had to call the police. Another time when I went to the chemist to get his medication, I phoned home, and when he answered, he said he had just knocked his dad out. He has pulled a knife on me. I don't get frightened. I keep seeing him as the little boy I used to bath and put to bed. He's my son – I can't be frightened of him, but I'm frightened of him for other people. I'm fearful for his dad. My son can't control his anger. We've had to call the police three or four times; we're really struggling. I'm exhausted, because he still doesn't sleep a proper night, and then it can be a three-hour battle to get him out of bed in the morning.

'We applied for a residential place, but by the time the authority agreed, they could not cope with his needs. His behaviour has escalated and he's lost routine. At the moment, he is not in school and a support worker is looking after him at home.

'Work has been my saving grace; it's the one thing I feel I am quite good at. At home, you lose your sense of self. I've become conditioned to battle. I'm not the easy-going person I could have been or should have been. Time and again, I have been let down or betrayed by professionals I thought I could trust.

'There was one day when I was heading home and I was going to take a bottle of paracetamol. I'd had enough. That's not me – I'm a strong person, but I feel I've got nowhere with the professionals. I don't mince my words, but I don't shout or swear. Last September I said to a social worker that I couldn't cope and if you don't help, I'm bringing him in and leaving him with you. They referred me to a panel hearing and we ended up getting two hours more respite-care a week.

'We're very isolated, because everyone keeps their distance, so thank you for listening. It's therapeutic. You know what you're experiencing is not normal, but by talking about it, you realize you have been through something unique.'

The loneliest and hardest fight for these mothers was the role they took on to defend the value of their child's life. After years of working with families and her own experience as the mother of an adult autistic son, one member of staff admitted some responses of professionals horrified her: 'I detect a view that they think these autistic children are getting a very high level of expensive care, and they question the point. Some seem to think that it's a waste, and that the lives of these children have no value. But whose life has value and by what measure?'

Care is where we make profound collective decisions about the worth of an individual life. If someone will never be employed, and will always be dependent on the care of others, are they of less value? To argue that market participation – earning and buying – is how we determine human worth is clearly objectionable. The great post-war achievement of the welfare state was its huge ambition, its universalism – all British citizens were eligible for care, and it offered comprehensive care throughout every stage of life. Compromises emerged early on; prescription charges and dentistry were early examples. Various forms of care, such as mental health, disability and the elderly, came to be known as the 'Cinderella services', because they were so poorly resourced, prompting a succession of politicians through the 1960s and 1970s to initiate urgently need reforms. The emergence of the disability-rights movement, inspired by US civil rights in the 1970s, shifted the public debate dramatically over the next twenty years, arguing for inclusion, specialist support, tolerance and adaptations to transport and the built environment. The campaigns and advocacy for disability won striking legislative victories.

The post-war ambition was the product of a remarkable moment of solidarity, born of a unique set of historical circumstances: two catastrophic world wars had undermined old class divisions, revealing common suffering. It generated a political commitment to the public services which lasted several decades, until the late 1970s. What followed was an erosion of that shared commitment; the individual was to be responsible for their own fate, and many forms of dependence came to be vilified. The values of the market infiltrated the language of worth and value. Solidarity became an old-fashioned notion. That leaves charities like the one I visited beleaguered outposts. They represent values which may win gestures of support intermittently – in politicians' speeches or fundraising initiatives – but not the long-term financial commitment to secure their own sustainability. Like thousands of other such small voluntary-sector organizations, it lurched precariously from grant to grant, badly hit by local-authority spending cuts. The significance of their work of solidarity, witness, advocacy and advice went beyond the lifeline it provided to a few hundred families. It was holding to an ideal. In the determined defiance of their remarkable stories, the staff and mothers were not just protecting their own children; they were asserting the value of being human, regardless of competence, skill and economic participation. At some point, we all end up on this battlefield, if only through the process of ageing, and their rallying cry is one on which many of us may come to depend.

Nine months later, the charity which arranged these interviews faced bankruptcy after a major grant-provider pulled out.
After a few months of uncertainty and a frantic scramble to keep
going, a third of the staff lost their jobs and it had to close down
its services in some cities.

(iii)

kindness

kindness, noun – state or quality of being kind.

kind, adjective – 1. Of a friendly, generous, benevolent or gentle nature. 2. Showing friendliness, affection or consideration.

The word 'kindness' has become a battle cry for humane public services. In *Intelligent Kindness*, John Ballat and Penelope Campling, who both have experience of working in the NHS, suggest that in healthcare they had a 'frequent sense that kindness is the junior partner alongside other ideologies and goals, leaning over the shoulder of more important things'. What was needed was 'to rescue the concept from the grip of a range of social and cultural forces that warp, denigrate and obscure what it is, marginalize kindness in the debate about what matters and make it more difficult to be kind'.

Kindness is often portrayed as something simple, straightforward and instantly recognizable. It is not as demanding as empathy, not as loaded with religious weight as compassion, and not contaminated like pity: no one could argue with the likeability of kindness; it represents something homely and uncontroversial in human relationships. But I am not convinced that kindness is easy or simple. It flows from a disposition, a way of seeing others. It's an expression of character, and of world view. It may become habit, it may be imitated, and it can even become convention, but it springs from powerful and deeply embedded histories of solidarity.

In their book *On Kindness*, the psychoanalyst Adam Phillips and the historian Barbara Taylor suggest that 'people are leading secretly kind lives all the time, but without a language in which to express this or cultural support for it'. An age-old confidence that people were naturally kind has evaporated. Instead, they argue that 'most people as they grow up now secretly believe that kindness is a virtue of losers' and that kindness has become 'incidental' and 'implausible'. Children need adults to help them 'discover and enjoy the pleasures of caring for others'.

Kindness is rooted in an Old English word, *cynde*, which carried meanings of something that was innate and natural as well as something that existed between kin. Kindness implied recognition of a common bond, a sense of belonging to each other; 'kindness is being in solidarity with human need', suggest Ballat and Campling.

I love how the kindness of a stranger acts like magic, transforming the moment. The pleasures of being kind were evident to the Stoics, who believed that kindness was the fount of happiness and that 'it expanded the soul'. Their emphasis on the pleasures of being kind was obscured by Christianity's preoccupation with self-sacrifice. Rousseau believed human beings were born instinctively kind, and this capacity for fellow feeling was the midwife to the development of the self, and could be crippled by civilization. But over the nineteenth century, the strand of thought which saw kindness as 'soft' and 'emotional' gained ground, and it became associated with femininity, while men were required to be public-spirited. Kindness became the pursuit of women, and was thus marginalized in public and professional life. Kindness needs to be rehabilitated.

Phillips and Taylor believe the impulse to be kind 'comes from the part of ourselves that we are most disturbed by, the part that knows how much assurance and (genuine) reassurance is required to sustain our sense of viability'. They conclude that 'it is kindness, fundamentally, that makes life seem worth living; and that everything that is against kindness is an assault on our hope'. Their argument was echoed in a blog by Jonathan Tomlinson, a GP working in the East End of London: 'We need institutions and cultures where people are kind to each other, where kindness is valued and nurtured in everything we do. Unless we are routinely subject to the kindness of others, we will have little kindness to share ourselves. The kindness of others sustains our own.'

4

Care as Dark Matter

IN THE HOSPITAL

'Compassion, the fairest associate of the heart.'

THOMAS PAINE,
'A Letter Addressed to the Abbe Raynal',
The Political Writings of Thomas Paine, 1824

My next journey took me to the other end of the country, to a busy teaching hospital where I was to shadow nurses and nursing assistants on a ward. In stark contrast to the charity's tiny offices, I was in a new, purpose-built hospital that reminded me of an airport, its corridors teeming with staff, patients and visitors. At the 7.30 a.m. handover meeting on the ward, the nurses crowded into the small staff room, mugs of tea or coffee in hand, to listen to the rattle of bed numbers, names, ailments, diagnostic procedures and discharge dates.

No other job is so clearly defined by care as nursing. The word litters a plethora of health policy documents, nurse training texts, inquiries, commissions and government reports. Experts expound on what it is for a nurse to provide care, how one does it, how organizations ensure it happens, and how nurses should be trained to provide it. The definitions have shifted dramatically since Florence Nightingale, the great Victorian reformer, first took up the task, and will continue to do so. There are good reasons for the interest. Nurses (predominantly women) are the backbone of the NHS, representing nearly a third of the clinical workforce (287,000). To a large extent, the quality of healthcare is in their hands. Unlike the last chapter's largely hidden crisis, here is one which is centre stage in public debate, subject to intense scrutiny and concern.

Nurses are on the front line of the increasing need for care. Demand on the NHS is rising sharply; in the decade to 2015/16, operations jumped by 40 per cent and hospital admissions by a third. Patients stay in hospital for shorter times (the average stay is now 7 days, compared to 10 days in France) and it becomes harder to develop relationships as the throughput of patients accelerates. There is constant pressure to reduce the Length of Stay figure, which is regarded as an easily measurable index of efficiency. The Department of Health uses it as a NHS performance indicator, with 'improvements' expected annually. In large part, the increase in hospital admissions reflects the ageing demographic, a growing population and the rise in long-term conditions, which by 2029 will affect 18 million, with a further 2.9 million suffering from multiple conditions. The main responsibility for managing this complex care will fall on nurses. Policy experts describe it as the 'carequake'.

But while need is growing, the number of nurses in the UK is falling. Overwork and low pay have damaged morale. More nurses are leaving the profession than are joining it, and vacancy rates were running at 12 per cent in 2019 – a total of 41,000 vacancies – leading to huge expenditure on agency fees to fill the gaps. Between 2009 and 2016 the ratio of nurses per 100,000 of the population dropped sharply in the UK, and is now almost half that in Sweden, Germany and France. Certain specialisms have been hit particularly hard in the last decade, such as learning disability (which fell by 41 per cent) and mental health (which fell by 10.6 per cent), despite increased need. Furthermore, the nursing workforce is ageing: 49 per cent of nurses were over 45 and only 24 per cent were under 34 in 2017. Retention and recruitment were badly damaged by below-inflation pay increases from 2010 to 2018. The scrapping of bursaries and introduction of tuition fees for nursing degrees in 2016 led to applications falling by a third. (Bursaries are due to be restored in 2020 but nurses will still have to pay £9,000 a year tuition fees.) On current trends, the NHS will have a shortfall of 108,000 nurses by 2029. The UK has traditionally relied on importing nurses, but after the Brexit referendum of 2016, the number of EU nurses registering to work in the UK fell by 96 per cent. With many developed countries needing more nurses, international competition for their crucial skills is sharp. As mentioned in Chapter 1, an alarmed House of Commons Select Committee on Nursing in 2018 urged that the 'nursing workforce needs to be expanded at scale and pace', and expressed 'concerns about the impact of pressures on morale, retention and standards of care'.

The dimension of the crisis uppermost in the public mind is that crucial aspects of care are being dangerously overlooked. The scandal of the Mid Staffordshire NHS Foundation Trust in the 2000s, when hundreds of patients were given 'appalling care' and many suffered, has left an enduring anxiety that the priorities of modern healthcare too often distort the role of nurses so that they cannot be attentive to the individual patient. Following the Francis report into the scandal, a raft of initiatives was launched to promote compassion. But as one report concluded, 'if finance and productivity are perceived as the only things that matter, it can have profound negative effects on the value placed on work as care-givers'; it feared that the job of nursing is 'increasingly protocol driven and reliant on technology ... [which] may have improved clinical effectiveness, but can be impersonal and lacking in compassion.' In 2012 the journalist Christina Patterson wrote a series of moving articles on care, which prompted an outpouring of responses from readers with similar experiences: 'I tried to explain what it feels like to be lying in a hospital bed in so much pain you can't even reach out for water, and feel that if you press your buzzer, you're going to make someone cross. I tried to explain what it feels like to hear the groans of people around you whose calls for help aren't being answered. And what it feels like to hear nurses who aren't even trying to whisper complaining about other patients, and you. I had never felt so abandoned or so alone.'

Nursing is a profession which has been profoundly shaped by the historic contradictions of care. Bedevilled by low pay and low status, nursing has struggled for autonomy and respect. Nurses have fought for a 'socially valued place and distinctive iden-tity' for over 150 years, Suzanne Gordon and Siobhan Nelson conclude in their influential and passionate book on the crisis. Nursing has been idealized, sentimentalized and vilified. Gosia Brykczynska sums up nursing's dilemma: 'the very familiarity contributes to its being undervalued and yet it is one of the most demanding interpersonal endeavours that can be undertaken and which is best accomplished when least noticed'. It straddles dualistic ways of thinking – reason or emotion, competence or compassion, efficiency or relationship. Good nursing requires all of these things, as Florence Nightingale well understood. But the remarkable persistence of her myth has done much damage to the profession she did so much to establish. In 1859 she wrote that the good nurse 'must make no demand upon the patient for reciprocation, for acknowledgement or even perception of her services; since the best service a nurse can give is that the patient shall scarcely be aware of any – shall perceive her presence only by perceiving that he has *no* wants'. This model of self-effacement has had a lasting legacy. A century later, the feminist writer Ann Oakley shamefacedly admitted that, after spending fifteen years as a sociologist studying medical services, she had been 'particularly blind to the contribution made by nurses'. She commented, 'I hardly noticed nurses at all. I took their presence for granted. And the character of the nurse's role in no way impressed itself on me.'

Gordon and Nelson argue that these exacting ideals 'leave nurses and nursing with no line of defence against the fiscal and economic rationalizers in healthcare'; historically, their work has been designed not to be noticed, to be taken for granted and to be subsidised by expectations of the nurse's goodness of heart.

Professor Alison Leary told me, 'Policymakers seem to find it very difficult to hear that they have to pay and educate to get the professional care which gets good outcomes. I've sat in meetings with civil servants and they still have an assumption that nursing is just about character, about being a nice person, and that it's all down to virtue.' On the day we met for our interview, Leary was exasperated by a storm on Twitter the previous evening over how the Universities and Colleges Admissions Service (UCAS) had defined nursing. 'It was all the old stereotypes about nurses as the handmaid of the doctor. It omitted to mention all the nurses in senior management positions, in public health and research. It was patronizing and plain wrong. Thankfully they have taken it down. But the prejudices about the role of the nurse are very entrenched.'

Anne Marie Rafferty, President of the Royal College of Nursing and Professor of Nursing Policy at King's College, London, has been at the forefront of nursing education for several decades. She admits her frustration at defining a nurse's care: 'Eighty percent of the universe is dark matter but scientists can't find it – it's the same with that ineffable part of care. It's just as big and just as hard to pin down.'

Derek sits in a chair beside his bed on the busy hospital ward. I'm shadowing Sam, the ward sister, who is accompanying the consultant, and several junior doctors, on his round. Derek looks up at the professionals standing around his bed. His hospital gown keeps slipping over his bare shoulder. He must be in his sixties, his white hair unkempt, and he strokes his beard repeatedly. He barely reaches five feet. His expression is almost childlike, and his eyes go through you. Wide open with anxiety, his forehead furrowed, he is beseeching someone – anyone – to help.

The consultant sits down on the bed and, without looking at Derek, turns to the two female junior doctors and rattles off acronyms and medical terms. He breaks off to make a swift comment to Derek: 'It's the alcohol.'

Derek protests, and tries to offer an explanation, but is cut off.

The consultant turns enquiringly to me, and Sam explains that I am shadowing her for the day. 'Sam is an excellent nurse, and it was obvious from the start. She had common sense,' he tells me, and then adds a startlingly inappropriate and untrue comment on her good looks: 'She's a part-time model.' Sam looks embarrassed.

Derek is looking from person to person, hoping for eye contact, for someone who might listen to him, but the consultant is reeling off instructions to Sam to ensure that Derek understands that he must take his medication. 'It's more important than anything I can do on the operating table,' he mutters on his way out.

Once he has gone, the work of nursing starts. Sam sits down, and places a hand on Derek's arm to try and calm his anxiety. Finally, he can start to explain. He has to get home. It's urgent. He looks after his mother. His sister lives several hundred miles away and they don't get on. The information comes in bursts.

'It's not the alcohol, it's that I had a riding accident, I fell off a horse and cracked my skull. I nearly died, I should have died. That's why I forgot to take the tablets.'

Sam listens, but she is also looking for a moment to interrupt, because she needs to find out why he forgets one of the four tablets he has to take every day.

'I'm not right. I've never been right. It's me that's the problem,' he says, his eyes filling with tears. 'I must get home. I've been in hospital twice in my life and both times I was under a death sentence. I need to get out of here.'

Sam tries to steer the conversation to blister packs. If his medication was allocated for each day, so that he just had to pop the blister and take the tablets inside, could he manage that? He nods, and begins to look less anxious. Once he has the blister pack, he can go home to look after his mother. He brightens, and even makes a joke: 'Give me a pill to die.' He laughs bleakly.

A blister pack seems a small thing. But it's an issue that runs through the rest of the day. It usually takes twenty-four hours to order – or more. Sam can't get hold of the pharmacist to speed up the process. She dashes to the hospital pharmacy to hand-deliver the order, only to discover it won't be ready until the following day.

Derek sits in his chair in his gown all day, staring miserably into space. The bed manager comes round in the afternoon, looking for beds; hospital occupancy is on red alert and she wants Derek's. Sam has had to explain first to Derek and then to the bed manager why he can't be discharged.

In between chasing the blister pack, Sam is looking after eight other patients and keeping an overview of the twenty-bed ward. She is on the move continuously. She started work at 7.30 a.m. and didn't get a chance to sit down until 1.40 p.m. for her forty-five-minute lunch break – six hours on her feet, with only the odd moment to grab a sip of water from her bottle.

One patient insists on choosing which nurses will attend to her. On this shift only Sam is allowed into her room. In addition, 'A4' is autistic and is proving challenging; patients are referred to by their bed number, a convenient form of shorthand between staff to swiftly locate the relevant patient, but it's disconcertingly impersonal. A few days before, A4 had threatened staff if they refused to take him out for a smoke. Now he is asking to be shaved; he wants his thick beard cut off. He needs clippers. He needs help with the phone call to the person at home who has the clippers. Sam makes the call, unsure if she will have time to shave him.

Every visit to the controlled medicine cupboard – several per hour – entails finding the one set of keys on the ward. They have to be passed back and forth between the qualified nurses dozens of times a day. I don't notice one moment of irritability.

Every hour, Sam has a form to fill in – ticking off a list of questions on pain, the availability of water, visits to the toilet – for each patient. When she is back at the computer, a list of icons flash to indicate tests and observations needed on each patient. The audit trail accompanies her all day – has she done everything she needs to do and has she done the paperwork to prove it?

Even towards the end of the punishing twelve-hour shift, Sam's tone and manner remain consistent and level. The same sing-song tone, determined cheerfulness and frequent endearments to colleagues and patients. 'Lovely' is the term Sam most often uses: 'All right, lovely?'

The hospital management has banned such terms of endearment, I was later told, but the ruling is ignored. Endearments ease the constant requests for help which characterize the interactions between nurses, because care is unpredictable, and suddenly several pairs of hands can be needed; a patient will need cleaning – there is blood or faeces everywhere – or another patient is deeply distressed. Responsibilities are shifted back and forth within the team.

It's like watching a piece of theatre. As Sam walks on to the ward, she assumes a role which matches the expectations placed on her by the patients to be kind, cheerful and calm. Another nurse referred to the performance as a 'front'. It's a mask which provides a professional identity and offers some personal protection from the emotional demands of individuals such as the pitiful Derek. The performance must never appear routine or automatic, and it requires constant adaptation to the needs of each patient. As with acting, the performance requires a giving of self to the role. Yet, unlike an actor's, this performance denies it is such; nurses are expected to be 'genuine' and 'human' – without the human traits of impatience or irritability. Nurses are subject to a powerful projection: to be ideal humans. Coping with this idealization is part of the job.

There were moments when their work showed the strain they were under and I saw it as less genuine, more performance. The head cocked to the side to denote sympathy, the hand on the arm, the sing-song tone, the 'take care', the endearments; more seriously, communication could slip when the nurse was not listening carefully enough, attempting to finish the patient's sentence or interrupt to speed up the point, their mind in too many other places.

As we race downstairs and along corridors, again in pursuit of the blister pack, Sam answers questions: 'I cope by going home and offloading on my husband. He's a delivery driver. He doesn't always understand, but he listens and that helps me put things into perspective. He has lost several members of his family to cancer.

'Sometimes when I start crying, I can't stop, so I hold it back. When my father-in-law died, I felt I had to suck it in, and play a containing role for my husband. Sometimes it's really stressful and my heart is palpitating, but I say to myself, deal with it, and it eases off.

'I suppose by "suck it in" I mean a kind of acceptance and determination: it will pass. When my grandma was ill with cancer and didn't have long to live, I had to sit my parents down and explain that she was dying. I felt I had taken on the adult role – the job they didn't want to do. I had to do the same with my father-in-law. If I am helping my parents and my husband, then I don't worry about myself.

'I absolutely love the job. I was in retail and I went into nursing as an auxiliary and I have worked my way up. I couldn't imagine doing anything else now.'

She is exceptionally conscientious, and I ask if she ever says no to a patient's request.

'I know some nurses won't help with some things – like shaving or making a call – but that's not my way. Besides, there is always the danger that someone will complain. Yes, there have been complaints. Someone might complain that a patient didn't have enough water on a particular day, but how do I explain that it was such a difficult day that I didn't have a chance to drink?'

Emotion breaks through at unexpected moments on the job. Tim is about to be discharged after a broken leg. He is over eighty but in good health, and patiently waits to be picked up. As we stand by the bed, he explains how he was out walking alone when he fell, and how the paramedics stretchered him off the narrow country path. His wife died a few months ago, sixteen weeks after she was diagnosed with a rare cancer. They had scattered her ashes on a favourite beach. He is a dignified man with a quiet cheerfulness, and this sudden set of confidences is overwhelming. Later, his daughter and grandchild pick him up, and he smiles and waves goodbye as he is wheeled out. Both Sam and I blink back tears. The tragedies are compressed – a few sentences or a gesture – and frequent, as human dramas are played out of love and loss, death and life, daily. Our tears are as much about the evident warmth of his family as the tragedy he has confided. Three generations discuss the apple trees he needs to prune while his daughter pushes him out of the ward. Hospitals are alive with snapshots of lives at moments of crisis and vulnerability.

Beneath the purposeful rush of staff, the worried relatives, and the anxious patients, is the steady beat of fear in the hospital; the corridors, wards and waiting rooms are thick with the anticipation of threat and emotion. Staff have little time, patients have all the time, and the mismatched temporal experience provokes stress. Good care in such an environment is fragile, always in danger of being swamped by anxiety, and only sustained by the quality of staff relationships and inspirational leadership.

There are tubs of chocolates in the ward's windowless staff room and they empty over the course of the day – gifts from grateful patients and their relatives. The staff survive the long shifts on sweets and tea. A wall in the staff room is covered in thank-you cards: 'Amazing', 'Can't thank you enough', 'Incredible'.

Some of the old hands maintain that the patient-nurse relationship has changed. Patients are more assertive, they look it all up on Google, they challenge you on obscure hospital regulations. They click their fingers and get impatient. They threaten to sue, they make complaints. They forget that a nurse may have others to look after. There's a culture of entitlement; they've 'paid their National Insurance' and expect their money's worth. Some families drop off their elderly relatives before they go on holiday. 'Us nurses are expected to cope and put up with it,' one nurse grumbled in the staff room in a break. I noticed that the only person on the ward to use the word thank you was Tim, but when I ask, Sam says she doesn't think they should be thanked.

The shift is almost done. I overhear Sam making yet another call about the blister pack. She is still calm. It's the first time I have seen her sitting down since her lunch break, and it is now past seven in the evening, yet I'm told it has been a quiet day. The previous week they had been short-staffed, and had six patients with dementia, several of whom were wandering around the ward, confused. Staff referred to such days as a 'war zone', and they fear making a disastrous mistake under the pressure.

After Sam finishes her call, I get a chance to ask what she had thought of the consultant's comment about her being a part-time model. It had made her feel uncomfortable, she admitted, and shrugged her shoulders. It's 8 p.m. and she has to drive home, kiss her eighteen-month-old baby good night and be back on duty the following morning at 7.30 p.m. There is no time to dwell on it.

In the last thirty years, the work of nurses has changed dramatically. The starched uniforms and elaborate codes of belts, badges, caps and dresses denoting a strict hierarchy have all been swept away; many of the nurses I shadowed wore what was described as pyjamas – a much cheaper form of clothing, confessed the hospital's director of nursing. More importantly, the bulk of the day-to-day work, known as 'basic care' – feeding, washing and help with the toilet – once the main component of a nurse's job, is now done by healthcare assistants or nursing auxiliaries. Sometimes they have had only a few weeks' training. As healthcare has become more technical, with frequent diagnostic procedures and specialists to coordinate, the nurse's attention has moved to the computer screen and the telephone. Their role is one of coordination, planning, liaison and discharge. Particularly the last, as Sam's struggle with the blister pack demonstrated; the pressure to free up beds is intense and becomes one of the main preoccupations of ward sisters, as hospitals clock up record occupancy levels. The number of hospital beds has declined and, with increased admissions, occupancy reached an average of 88 per cent in 2019. Anything over 85 per cent is dangerous, warns the National Institute of Clinical Excellence, leading to bed shortages and periodic crises.

Healthcare assistants are increasingly taking on even medical tasks (with appropriate training), such as cannulation (inserting a tube into a vein to allow for intravenous drugs), catheterization (the insertion of a tube to drain the bladder), dressing wounds and taking blood. It is estimated that only 40 per cent of a nurse's time on average is spent directly with patients, and some studies put the figure much lower. Nurses talk of their task of 'hunting and gathering' to find equipment and chase test results. One policy report described their task as 'the common denominator along the care pathway'.

There is deep unease about this shift amongst both nurses and the general public. Debbie Field, a consultant nurse at London's Royal Brompton Hospital, commented at a conference, 'the word "basic" is used in a meaningless way. To distinguish between basic and professional nursing care is a false dichotomy, the two are inseparable; turning, bathing, mouth care all have value, because they provide an opportunity to connect with the patient, to get to know them, and be with them. It is basic in the true sense of the word, as the fundamentals of nursing care.' The fear amongst patients and relatives is that as nursing moves away from the bedside, it becomes impersonal. 'The loudest message we heard from the public was that there were too few nurses and they did not have enough time to care. Typical concerns included not being able to dedicate more time to caring and actually knowing their patients,' commented a report on the future of nursing. Another report warned that 'as nursing becomes more academic, old values may have slipped away. Basic care is delegated to staff with the least qualifications and lowest status, by implication, spending time with patients is devalued.'

But others in the profession celebrate that nurses are finally being liberated from the historic position of 'handmaid' to the doctor. In the past, nothing more was expected of a nurse than to be hardworking and kind. Now nursing degrees at universities bring prestige to the profession in its long battle for recognition in the doctor-dominated healthcare system. With higher nursing qualifications comes greater autonomy, the authority to diagnose and prescribe medication and lead clinical teams. These new roles are welcome progress for ambitious nurses, but it leaves nagging concerns.

'There is a depersonalization and we touch less. When I was a front-line nurse, I would hold patients who were distressed,' said the director of nursing at Sam's hospital, reflecting on her thirty-year career. She admitted that nursing was changing: 'Recently I saw someone wearing gloves to wash a patient and I asked why – there was no good clinical reason. I think they saw it as some form of barrier. A year ago, when visiting a ward, I saw a nurse who was sitting on the bed, and she jumped up and said, "Sorry, I was just talking." She felt she had to apologize. Perhaps we don't value relationship enough, socially and culturally.'

The management models imported into healthcare from business in the last thirty years have contributed to these trends. The focus has been on efficiency, productivity and financial controls; in successive waves of controversial healthcare reform, areas of the NHS have been restructured to open up competition in services, carving out areas such as cleaning and diagnostics for privatization. Commercial interests have eroded the ethos of public service. A new language has infiltrated every corner of healthcare, in which staff are instrumentalized as a means to an end, be that balanced budgets or targets for waiting times. One report referred to the 'size of the spend' on nurses' wages, suggesting that 'we simply do not know whether the public gets the best return on this investment and whether the potential of nursing and midwifery capital is fully exploited'.

Human beings were comparable to a financial asset. Energetic macho verbs proliferate: 'driving up' standards; 'waging war' on obesity; the 'fight' against cancer. This issue was identified in 2013 in the influential Francis Inquiry Report into the scandal of the Stafford Hospital run by the Mid Staffordshire NHS Foundation Trust; one of its conclusions was that the board's preoccupation with organizational change and meeting national targets for finance and waiting times had compromised the quality of care. It called for a renewed commitment to compassion as the foundation of nursing. But despite the attention the inquiry received, concern persisted that the way healthcare was being commercialized damaged care. In an article in the *BJPsych Bulletin* in 2016, Penelope Campling suggested that promoting a competitive market economy in health led to a 'commodified view of need, skills and service', and warned that it 'insidiously affects the attitudes, feelings and relationships of staff'. She argued that the emphasis on regulation and performance management had led to processes and systems dominating the workload. 'Not everything can be counted, described, scientifically analysed,' Gordon and Nelson conclude in their study of nursing, and they fear that the dominance in healthcare of a scientific, objective model can only ever trivialize care and risk losing it in a 'sea of saccharine'.

Professor Alison Leary's concern is that the wrong things get measured, leading to 'pointless tickbox routines'. One of the recommendations of the Francis Inquiry Report is a case in point, she adds. 'Intentional rounding' requires the nurse to check on every patient every hour and fill out a form (as I observed Sam do). It was a measure intended to 'mitigate skills dilution on the ward' (resulting from the use of healthcare assistants), she explains, 'but the evidence of a major research project is that it has no effect. Plenty of nurses pointed that out long ago but their voice is not listened to. They don't have the authority required to get the point across. It's a misogynistic bias against nurses. Look at the research on safe staffing – 700 papers proving that if you cut staff, people die. I stand in front of NHS boards and tell them not to reduce staff. They listen to me because I'm a mathematician and a computer scientist and I put up some equations on a projector, but I'm only saying the same thing as their director of nursing.'

Leary's first career was as an engineer, and she draws comparisons with nursing. Both deal with risk. 'As an engineer, I was socialized to accept that there is always risk, and your role is to understand the risk and mitigate it. Good care is always managing risk. In healthcare, the stakes are high, but the culture around risk is very different. We can't tolerate it, and everyone is always trying to eliminate it, which is not honest. When there is a problem in the airline industry, people analyse the situational context, staffing levels, etc. All factors are relevant, but in healthcare it always comes back to the question of character and apportioning blame to individuals. "Bad apple" is the commonest strategy, but invariably the problem is systemic.'

The following day, I was back at the hospital on the oncology ward to shadow a healthcare assistant, John, and an auxiliary, Sally. By the time I arrived at nine o'clock, they had been at work for two hours, serving breakfast and helping people wash. The curtains had been pulled around the family of a dying man. Others lay on their beds, very ill and barely speaking, except to answer questions briefly. They had only months to live, and much of that time was likely to be spent coming in and out of this ward. But John and Sally wanted me to understand that this was not a sad place. People might be dying, but their work was punctuated by smiles, laughter and jokes. As they arrived at the patient's bedside, they insisted that they gave them a smile. Their warmth and good intentions were evident, and most patients were persuaded to comply. A few enjoyed the jokes.

'They want to chat. They get so much information about the cancer and the treatment and its side effects. They get sympathy from family and friends. With us, they want to be normal,' John said.

Sally and John were responsible for many of the routine tasks once done by nurses. It was time for one man's wash and Sally persuaded him that he needed to get out of bed. He was patronizing, irritable and quick to find fault, but she humoured him, coaxing him into his chair. She spent about fifteen minutes encouraging him to wash himself, in line with new directives to encourage independence in patients. Meanwhile, John was comforting a confused and very distressed woman. 'I don't know why I am here,' she sobbed, 'I don't know what's wrong with me. Where is my son?' John calmed her down. As he took blood from her, he skilfully drew her into conversation. She had been a bank manager's secretary and '*very* efficient', she said with a fierce grimace, and then she was laughing. John had the bloods he needed for tests and he had his smile. She joked that ever since her divorce thirty-five years ago, she had had no use for men.

John and Sally in their routine work contained the unpredictable, the chaotic, the unruliness of emotions and bodies. A ward sister told me that part of her role was to remain calm. 'Care is about order and organization,' she said. 'One needs to contain the complexity, and that instils confidence in staff, the patients and their relatives. At a point of crisis, patients and relatives are often out of control, and there is an unspoken ask: please take control.'

In the bed next to the confused woman, Harry, a truck driver, had barely said a word all morning. Divorced, and unsure about the whereabouts of his four children, he had lung cancer. He had come to live with his sister while he was being treated.

John struggled to get a smile. Harry's cancer was terminal. The silences were painful.

John has been a healthcare assistant for over fifteen years, and was paid £10 an hour: £19,000 a year. He has to top up his wages with a Sunday shift at the supermarket, but he was very upset that the overtime payments which made that worthwhile were being phased out. Before nursing, he had worked full time at the supermarket, and still had the task of cutting cold meats for the start of the week. As I watched him take blood, admit patients to the ward and fill in the paperwork, I thought about his six-day week to make ends meet. John left home at 6.15 a.m. for a 7 a.m. start, and did not finish his shift until 7.30 p.m. Nursing is a very physical job, requiring huge amounts of energy. John nipped back and forth, picking up equipment, dropping off things, filling in forms, changing beds, handing out food. In one cupboard, he showed me a hair dryer.

'We always pair up to lay out the dead. We wash and dry the body and the hair. Relatives don't want to see their loved one with greasy hair. We always talk to the dead person as if they were alive. We open the window to let the soul out.'

There is a big round sticker on every ward door. Around the edge, the six Cs of nursing – *care, compassion, competence, communication, courage* and *commitment* – and in the centre, the slogan, 'Care is our business.' Sally lamented that 'It's all just a business to those up at the top. But to me it's not. It's about people.' Sally saw this sticker and its attempt to explain her work dozens of times a day. To be true to the values which sustained her work, she quietly ignored some of the directives, such as the ban on endearments. She had a set of values which she did not believe were shared by the institution – a low-level conflict which coloured her working life.

In the ward's supplies cupboard, everything was labelled with a price: £16 for one dressing; 42p for another. The price of some of the chemotherapy injections was enormous. 'One injection can be £25,000. We're cheap in comparison,' said John. Money rankles. 'We're just a number. They'll string you up if you have a sick day. A staff nurse starts on £11 an hour after three years of university – the same as a junior manager at Aldi, yet we are dealing with people's lives.'

The word 'nurse' has origins in the French and Latin words meaning to nourish. It was originally used to describe breast-feeding. A woman nursed her child or handed her over to a wet nurse, hence its close association with women. The word carries the association of physical closeness; we may talk of someone who nurses a small bag on their lap, or a glass of brandy. It speaks of attentiveness and a slow pace. Historically, most nursing was the responsibility of the women of the family: wives, daughters and mothers. Best known of all Florence Nightingale's books is the bestselling *Notes on Nursing*, published in 1859, and a cheaper edition, *Notes on Nursing for the Laboring Classes*, was widely distributed in a bid to improve standards of care in the home. Nightingale wrote: 'Every woman in England has, at one time or another of her life, charge of the personal health of somebody, whether child or invalid – in other words, every woman is a nurse. How immense and valuable would be the produce of her united experience if every woman would think how to nurse.' Harriet Martineau, the American writer, described Nightingale's book as a 'work of genius', because 'the very elements of what constitutes good nursing are as little understood for the well as for the sick'.

Nightingale, who was intensely religious, was well aware that tending to the sick was a clear injunction of Christianity; the Sermon on the Mount specified visiting the sick as an act of charity – the requirement to show solidarity came before the capacity to ease suffering. In *Persuasion* Jane Austen describes

Nurse Rooke as someone whose conversation is 'entertaining
and profitable, something that makes one know one's species
better'. With little useful medical knowledge at the time, the
task of tending the sick was largely a matter of good company
and distraction. It was a point powerfully made in the recol-
lections of Walt Whitman, the American poet, on his work in
Washington's makeshift hospitals during the American Civil
War. Thousands of wounded young soldiers were pouring into
the city, and Whitman took it upon himself to invent his own
form of nursing care. With no medical training but plenty of
insight, creativity and dedication, he spent three years in the
crowded wards of military hospitals. 'To many of the wounded
and sick, especially the youngsters, there is something in personal love, caresses, and the magnetic flood of sympathy and
friendship, that does, in its way, more good than all the medicine
in the world … Many will think this merely sentimentalism,
but I know it is the most solid of facts. I believe that even the
moving around among the men, or through the ward, of a hearty,
healthy, clean, strong, generous-souled person, man or woman,
full of humanity and love, sending out invisible, constant currents thereof, does immense good to the sick and wounded.'

He prepared for each visit 'as carefully as a general prepares
for battle', writes his biographer, taking gifts, food and paper, so
that he could write letters for patients to their relatives. Above
all, he was stirred by the anonymity – what he described as
the 'obscurity' – of the suffering of these young men, and saw
his writing as a vocation 'to give identity to the lives of these
neglected and anonymous young men … My custom is to go
through a ward, or a collection of wards, endeavouring to give
some trifle to each, without missing any. Even a sweet biscuit, a
sheet of paper, or a passing word of friendliness, or but a look or
nod, if no more. In this way I go through large numbers without
delaying, yet do not hurry. I find out the general mood of the

ward at the time; sometimes see that there is a heavy weight of listlessness prevailing, and the whole ward wants cheering up. I perhaps read to the men, to break the spell … Every one of these cots has its history – every case is a tragic poem, an epic, a romance, a pensive and absorbing book, if it were only written.'

A few years earlier, Florence Nightingale had famously embarked on a similar task in the hospitals of the Crimea, where the British army was fighting Russia. Leading a group of a few dozen women, Nightingale attempted to bring comfort to the young soldiers. Contrary to the Nightingale myth, the women were allowed to do little more than help turn the patients, fan them in the heat and put ice in their mouths. Physical contact with the bodies of the young male soldiers was considered unacceptable. These well-meaning ladies were known as 'sympathizers'. Most of the actual nursing in the Crimea was done by the usual combination of wives, servants and orderlies, but a 'few well-born ladies' took the credit. Nightingale as the 'Lady with the Lamp' was a propaganda tool for a British government deeply embarrassed by the incompetence of the military – a useful distraction and a symbol of elite concern for the suffering ordinary soldier. But the mythology allowed a breakthrough in the development of nursing. Nightingale used it for her own reforming ambitions, and she succeeded in recasting nursing as a moral vocation for women.

In the mid-nineteenth century, as Nightingale prepared her reform plans, hospitals were places of dread, only used by the desperate, and typically more than half their occupants died of infection. One of the most famous literary portrayals of a nurse is Sarah Gamp in Charles Dickens' *Martin Chuzzlewit*: she was slovenly, almost continuously drunk, and intent on unscrupulous money-making. In stark contrast, Nightingale defined the profession according to Christian ideals. She was strongly influenced by the models of nursing developed in religious contexts in France and Germany, where one of the main tasks was to offer spiritual solace to the patient. In particular, Nightingale drew on the work of Saint Vincent de Paul's Daughters of Charity, founded in 1617; its members were allowed to leave the cloisters of the convent and visit the poor who were sick in their homes. This was radical for two reasons: it gave women an unusual degree of autonomy, and they were exposed to an intimate knowledge of others' bodies. To allay anxieties about their relative independence, great emphasis was laid on their virtue and their obedience to the religious order. Their work 'occurred wholly within a framework of submission, obedience and indifference ... religious orders demanded that nurses not only cultivate knowledge but also anonymity, and that they sacrifice every shred of their individual identity ... they gave up their given names, and adopted new ones assigned by the community'.

Similarly, Nightingale's nurses were to be selflessly dedicated to service, and obedient both to senior nurses and to doctors. In time, nurses came to be known as 'sisters', their uniforms were like those of nuns, and nurses' homes were run with strict bedtimes, like convents. Nightingale was creating a form of respectable paid employment for women – one of the first – and to do that, she shrewdly emphasized traditional gender stereotypes. An article in *The Times* shortly after her departure for the Crimea in 1854 talked of her womanly virtues, praising her for the charitable impulse which saw her quit 'the family circle which her taste and talents made her so fit to adorn'; other articles stressed her domesticity. The image was of an efficient housewife compelled by religious duty to apply her skills to the new environment of a hospital.

She created a profession which reflected her religious beliefs. There had long been a link between the gentlewoman's duty to visit the sick and proselytizing with religious pamphlets

(by the end of the nineteenth century, half a million women
volunteered for such work, and no doubt many were carrying
Nightingale's *Notes on Nursing*). Nightingale saw nursing as
having a moralizing mission at a time of great social change. She
also recognized, despite her own very privileged background,
women's desperate need for respectable employment, and she
ensured nursing was seen as 'an avenue of honest work'; but
to win this new opportunity for independence, women had to
conform to what is known as the 'moral script' of nursing.

What was concealed in this public-relations exercise was
Nightingale's remarkable skills as a statistician, sanitary reformer,
architect, lobbyist and writer. Although the Lady with the Lamp
became the myth, the reality was not a woman wandering around
the wards late at night to bring a gentle word to patients, but
a relentless researcher and politician. One admiring hospital
administrator in the Crimea said Nightingale had 'all the softness
and gentleness of her sex, all the cold clear-headedness of the
Mathematician, a capital head for devising ten thousand little
details of administration, and a resolute boldness that quails
before no obstacle'. Elizabeth Gaskell wrote a detailed account
of spending a few days with the great national icon; at first deeply
impressed, she described her as a 'saint, completely led by God',
but her admiration waned as she detected the steeliness: 'she
does not care for individuals – but for the whole race of God's
creatures'. They had a 'grand quarrel' over the need to visit a poor
neighbour; Nightingale declared she was too busy with plans
for a hospital. 'She is too much for institutions, sisterhoods and
associations,' wrote Gaskell, after Nightingale told her that 'if she
had children, she would send them all to a well-managed creche
and would expect all mothers to do likewise.'

But none of this emerged in public. Nightingale's challenge
was to pioneer a role for women without antagonizing the powerful medical lobby. It came at the cost of any claim to authority,

leadership or status. At the same time, she ensured the feminization of nursing. Whitman's account is a reminder of traditions of male nursing, particularly amongst all-male communities, such as the military and monastics, but little of its legacy is left in modern nursing. The moral script requiring a virtuous and generous femininity persists and nurses are expected to 'go the extra mile', to be uncomplaining and to be motivated by kindness rather than financial reward or recognition. Nurses have struggled to escape this gilded cage ever since.

Professor Anne Marie Rafferty has wrestled with this historical legacy throughout her career. She was amongst the first cohort to do a nursing degree in the UK in the late 1970s: 'We were being trained to be missionaries – or at least reformers – to be clever *and* to care. We were taught that our job was to analyse, critique and be agents of change: we had to use our brains. We were charged with a kind of iconoclasm to tear down the institutional structures on which nursing relied for its legitimacy. The status quo had to change – care had become routinized and ritualized. The role of the nurse was unquestioning of authority. They didn't exercise leadership and had neither the strength nor power to produce high quality care.

'We were told that pockets of poor care needed to be uprooted and a change was needed in the mindset and attitude of the profession. We were to be research-informed. It was a kind of cultural revolution in nursing. Instead of "custom and practice defines care", we were taught the application of the scientific method. The evaluation cycle mapped on to nursing: do an assessment, formulate a plan, then evaluate its success.

'My research shows that better educated nurses equals better nurses. This was the struggle we had to ensure all nurses took degrees. The media coverage played into the old stereotypes, with headlines such as 'Too posh to wash'. Instead of building on nursing degrees, skills are being diluted, with the growing use of healthcare assistants and now nursing apprentices. But we need highly educated nurses at every level. Nursing always seems to be on the back foot, and embattled; there are seventeen royal medical colleges for doctors and only one for nurses in the UK.'

The 'six Cs' I noticed in the hospital have been a source of deep frustration. They are viewed as both patronizing and reducing care yet again to an achievement of character. They include the 'competence' needed by nurses, but there is no acknowledgement of the expertise often required or the role of critical thinking. One of the difficulties, Rafferty points out, is the enormous complexity in the patient-nurse relationship: 'At its heart, nurses are always rationing effective engagement – that is the essence of good nursing. They need to ensure enough attention to satisfy need, but not too much to deprive another patient. It is stressful – you don't have time to deal with everything. There is always the unfinished emotional business of the relatives and the patient. You have to live with that tension and terror, and wrestle with it. The tension is even more prominent now because expectations about care – such as warmth, communicating, listening – are rising.

'Compassion can be squeezed out when the workload is excessive and you get burnout because you know you are not matching up to your own ideals. The historical construction of nursing has been idealized from the beginning; according to that, nurses are expected to give unstintingly of themselves. There is a strong Christian ethos which still runs through nursing. But compassion follows the right working conditions – it's a function of an environment, it's not an individual character trait. It's like a phenotype: the potential is there, but the genes only switch on in the right environment. If people don't have time, you sap morale and motivation.'

Interviewing nurses, I often sensed that descriptions of

their work left gaps, and fell short of conveying what Rafferty referred to as the 'power of nursing'. Rafferty's metaphor of care as the 'dark matter' of nursing began to make sense; much of what a nurse does has an invisibility. One A & E nurse jokingly acknowledged that while she talks to her husband a lot about her job and relies hugely on his support, she can't tell him about the 'blood and gore'. I noticed a slight hesitation as nurses assessed what level of detail I could tolerate. Nurses work with bodies which have become unruly and unpredictable; they clean up the piss, blood, phlegm, vomit and faeces. They know that these bodily secretions and their smells provoke anxiety, fear and revulsion. They develop a relationship with the body not required in other walks of life: a practical familiarity with its creases and folds, its orifices and secretions. They have an intimacy with skin, the biggest organ containing all others, and how it breaks down, how it heals, and how, through touch, it provides a form of powerful communication. Their work requires a constant crossing of the conventional boundaries of privacy, and it is the hands (literally) of the nurse which maintain the patient's dignity and respect. Their work contains and orders the materiality of bodies, an aspect of human experience which is profoundly disturbing. This task has always been a challenge, but even more so when most people have little experience of this aspect of the body. As care has been professionalized and largely removed to hospitals, people rarely handle physical decay and disease. Nurses are caught in a complex bind, helping us to forget or ignore something that they cannot. After they clean up a patient, overcoming or concealing their own sense of revulsion, they dismiss or make light of what they have done: 'It's nothing.'

The protection of a patient's dignity is a subtle interplay of both distance and reassurance. One nurse said he avoided eye contact when he was bathing a patient as a way of respecting their sense of dignity; only when he finished did he look them in the eye. On the wards, I noticed bathing or moving a patient in the bed was often accompanied by cheery comments; their purpose was to establish a sense of normality. Discussing the weather or where the patient lived were the everyday details which could reorientate them in the midst of the bewildering experience of a stranger washing their body. A nursing intervention can be a simple task, but can entail great skill. 'Professionalization of caring must never obscure the ordinariness and naturalness of [care]. The more we understand about caring, the better we shall be able to promote this ordinary yet ennobling and creative art,' writes Brykczynska. The conversation of the mental-health nurse with a patient may seem no more than casual chat, but it allows a process of assessment. The nurse in a GP surgery who jokes about the weather and going on holiday, builds trust, encouragement and a relationship. At the same time, they are able to interweave crucial information and make assessments.

One nursing academic described a disabled patient who did not have the capacity to hold a pudding plate still, and how the nurse, without comment, pushed the plate into place. Dignity was protected. In another example, a patient had spilled a urinal in the bed and needed cleaning. He was extremely embarrassed and felt humiliated, but 'the nurse's practised, gentle style rehumanized me'. When he thanked her a few weeks later, 'she didn't seem to understand the passion behind his praise'.

No other profession routinely belittles its own work. Self-deprecation was often commensurate with the enormity of the suffering a nurse was witnessing. Gilly, a senior Accident and Emergency nurse, described an occasion when a young man had died soon after being brought into the hospital. When the distraught mother arrived, Gilly arranged for the body to be moved to a side room where the mother could sit with her son. She stayed all night, and Gilly occasionally put her head round the door to check on her. In the morning, the mother said she had given her 'precious hours with her son', yet Gilly insisted to me it was 'a little thing'. In another example, Gilly accompanied a lady with a gynaecological emergency. 'She was barely conscious, and I kept talking to her as she went straight up to theatre. A few days later, I visited her on the ward, and she recognized my voice, and thanked me for holding her hand on the way to the theatre. I'm acutely aware that human touch and voice stay with people.'

Gilly acknowledged such gestures could be powerful, even transformative. 'We are very privileged when we share with somebody on a level they have never been to before. They have ultimate trust in you and you can give them some comfort at that time. We share people's most raw emotions, and for another human being to allow you to do that – well, it's a form of privilege.'

'Trust is very important. You pull on whatever is in you to quickly build it. If it's a kid, you might tell a joke. You have to work out if someone would appreciate a touch on the arm or not. Some people like to be called by their first name, some don't. How can I engage and make contact so that someone knows they are safe and we are listening to them? It is so important, because what happens in hospital is invasive and people can be in pain or feel vulnerable and anxious.'

Serving as a witness to another person's pain, and providing some relief, can be immensely powerful, affirming of one's own humanity, Gilly explained. At the same time, it can be humbling. 'Nurses are still the profession most trusted by the public in polls. That is such a privilege,' a hospital director of nursing said. 'People have divulged things to me which they told me they had never said to anyone else. Part of the expectation is that a nurse won't flinch. They are like shock absorbers, and they understand the need for confidentiality.'

The management theorist Valerie Isles makes a distinction

between 'simple, hard' and 'complex, easy' in the activities of an organization. The latter is more abstract, and relies on data and analysis. The former entails conversations and relationships which can be very difficult. Much of nursing falls into the 'simple, hard' category. Suzanne Gordon, the historian of nursing, warns that 'when efficiency is pursued through the gathering and measuring of data, the invisibility or "softness" of care makes it doubly disadvantaged. A false dichotomy emerges between care as emotional, relational and routine, while medicine acquires status as scientific, objective and rational.' She argues that there is a 'broad social failure to understand what nurses do embedded in the medical system ... which saps nurses' self-esteem, subjects them to disregard, disdain and outright abuse, and aggravates class and status dilemmas.'

On my last day shadowing nurses, I joined Pete, a community nurse, on his round of visits. In many ways he represents the future of nursing: taking care out of hospitals and helping the elderly, the chronically ill and the dying to remain at home for as long as possible. He went into nursing after working in air traffic control; my initial surprise at this career move gave way to seeing some parallels between the two forms of work. Both require coordinating complex activity.

'Care takes a lot of sorting out. I have to order a bed this afternoon and will have to fill out a form, add a covering letter and so forth. These kinds of bureaucratic tasks can't be delegated, because medical knowledge is needed to identify the right mattress. Not even ordering things like incontinence pads is straightforward – it has to be done through one of five 'pathways', but none of them apply in this case, so I will have to add a covering note. Paperwork can take hours. I'm pulled in every direction: there's my code of conduct as a registered nurse, in which I must be the patient's advocate, but that can come into conflict with the pressure to ration care. We invariably run into complex cases. Currently I have a case in which the daughter lives at the other end of the country and her mother is very sick. If the mother is moved to a home near the daughter, is her care funded from here or there? Two health trusts are now fighting it out through the courts, and it is all hinging on my initial decision as to why I sent her into respite care.'

Every aspect of his work is shaped by technology. 'A computer programme calculates "capacity" in our team; we have to log who we are seeing, travel times and administrative tasks continually. It then works out what capacity we are running at – it's usually 105 per cent, and that's red; it should be well below that to ensure spare capacity for emergencies. There are audit tools which monitor us washing our hands, how many of our elderly patients have had a fall, how many have had a catheter. We have to upload all that data. I have to input the times of visits with a cost of £28 each – they use those figures for the budget.'

A few months later, I shadowed Jack, a nurse in a GP practice. This is another form of the future of nursing; much of Jack's job is taken up with monitoring patients with long-term conditions. He fills in templates on the computer, taking blood pressure, blood and sputum samples. His screen had a tab for 'payment indicator', and he referred to 'making money for the practice'. The marketization of healthcare shaped how he understood his work, and the patient had become a means to 'make money'. But Jack ensured that the relationship remained central. At every appointment he managed to find a joke to make the patient smile. His quick one-liners and repartee put people at ease. It seemed effortless and casual, but it was neither. Every conversation was an opportunity to gather information about how patients were coping with complicated regimes of different inhalers and medication. He liked the routine nature of this job. But the level of data management – collection and processing – can easily dominate the interaction. Screening programmes require the participation of millions of people. The 'industrialization' of healthcare follows its own imperatives, in which the patient can be grist to the mill of data gathering.

While I shadowed these nurses, I saw the intense pressure they were under and their skill in focussing on the patient. They managed a delicate balance between efficiency and compassion, the ordinary and the extraordinary, the routine and spontaneity; their work required them to incorporate concepts usually regarded as opposites.

Tim, an intensive-care nurse in a major hospital, challenges many of the stereotypes, having done his first degree in engineering before embarking on a career in theatre. In his thirties he switched tack, but he sees a continuity between theatre and healthcare; both entail performance and story-telling, he suggested when we met in a pub for the interview. A powerful allegory for the direction his career has taken can be found in his work for Antony Gormley's Fourth Plinth project for Trafalgar Square in 2009, which entailed 2,400 people each spending one hour on the plinth over 100 days. Tim's role as event manager was to interview 500 applicants. 'I facilitated a significant moment in people's lives, and that's exactly what you get in nursing. Pursuing this interest in people's stories is the best part of nursing. When you can sit down and listen to someone. It's beautiful. What's exposed in a crisis is that fundamentally everyone is the same: everyone cares about themselves and about others. There is a lot of existential panic in hospitals, either from the fear of death or a threat to one's way of life and identity. In nursing that moment of opening up happens every day. It's routine. I saw lots of opportunities in nursing to explore those ideas, and to be with people in crisis, and help them at their most vulnerable. It's very human: trying to understand people, and understand my own humanity. I never stop learning.

'It's emotionally hard, seeing people who are incredibly upset for themselves and for others. But it is also very beautiful to see the love one person has for another. You don't see that much in everyday life. There are those moments when you get a lump in your throat. I know I'm opening up my life to others by spending time with them at their most vulnerable, and they are opening up to me. It's a shared journey and with that comes a real intimacy.

'In intensive care, one of the tasks is to keep explaining to the patient where they are, and who they are, to help them through the experience of delirium. I am repeating the same thing several times a day. 'It's Monday, the sun is shining, your partner is here. I am going to brush your teeth or wash you.' That kind of thing. I encourage the partners to speak to them too. It's a way of trying to draw them back.'

Tim brushed aside many aspects of nursing's troubled historical legacy. He has worked alongside a lot of other male nurses (they tend to cluster in intensive care and emergency medicine) and saw no difference in motivation or capability between men and women. Nor is he interested in the language of vocation. He acknowledges the work is very hard, physically demanding, with long shifts and barely time to drink enough water. He had to deal with things that made other people wretch – he cited a recent example of a patient with sepsis and how the pungent smell repulsed several nursing colleagues – but he insisted that the job was 'normal'.

I asked him what he meant by the word.

'A colleague saw someone die on an emergency ward and their response was that it was not normal. But death is normal. Tidying it away is not. Nurses are often very scared of death. They want a happy ending, and they want to make people feel better.'

'Normal' is a small, nondescript word for what Tim was describing: an existential recognition of how human bodies live, suffer and die. He maintained, furthermore, that the 'normal' response to suffering was to help: 'I think care is innate. You see it in children and amongst friends. You care for your family.' His parents have inspired his understanding of care, he told me; his mother was a nurse and his father a firefighter. 'After they've gone, you still care for your parents by remembering what they have taught you – that is a form of care. Honouring that lesson.' He was describing the art of care as an inheritance, a legacy from one generation to the next.

One of Tim's tutors was Ian Noonan, now Senior Lecturer in mental-health nursing at the University of Huddersfield. Like Tim, he saw the relationship between the arts and nursing, and used the analogy of music: 'I can almost hear the transposition from one key to another. I use music as a method of analysis: what is the underlying harmonic structure here? The art of nursing is a way of coming alongside someone. It's a form of improvisation, like jazz; it is flexible, responsive and co-creative. Art is not something you do to someone. At its best, it's a moment of grace.'

Ian's office was on a west-facing corner high above the street, and, as we talked, the sky reddened with a magnificent winter sunset. It was a fitting accompaniment to his language, but I was startled by the word 'grace'. He had started the interview with an emphatic declaration that it was bizarre the way nurses made care out to be something 'special and precious', which allowed them 'to be mystical about the work'.

'Grace?' I asked.

'Yes, that's the word. It's a really important idea. I'm not religious, but words such as "grace" and "service" are fundamental. Contemporary definitions of nursing care are too reductionist.

What about love – not romantic love, but agape? That's what drives nurses. Grace relates to placing someone else's needs before your own, but that is not about being a martyr, because it is so affirming of you. Grace is the fruit of care. Why should religion have all the best ideas? We can pinch them!' he said, laughing.

He offered an example from early in his training when he was twenty-one: 'I was working on a rehabilitation unit for people with severe and enduring mental illness. There was a woman who had been there a long time, and hadn't spoken coherently in years. As I walked past, I heard her hum something I recognized. I sat down with her and hummed the next line – it was from an opera. We spent twenty minutes humming together. Then she began to talk about an opera recording by Kathleen Ferrier, and how, as a child, she used to stay up to listen to it with her father. It was an incredibly moving moment. I felt a real joy to sit with her and to hold her hand. It was magical, a moment of grace and real pleasure.

'I think about care in nursing a lot, and the inadequacy of the language. Caring is an act of service, placing someone else's needs ahead of yours. It requires a constant process of analysis and reflection. It's the therapeutic use of self, not just seeing someone in an instrumental way as a means to an end.

'Defining care is hard – above all, you have to *do* things. There is always a danger of sentimentalization, and that is no use in nursing. Care must be about actions. My husband used to be a mental-health nurse, but he found the suffering overwhelming and left. I recognize that suffering, but I take the view that I can still make a cup of tea. I may not be able to sort it all out, but I can do something. The intervention can be modest, but I'm not diminished by that modesty – the cup of tea or the bed bath for faecal incontinence. The latter is more grim for the patient than for me. When they are clean and dry, I can sit down with them and talk.

'I remember at a homeless centre where I was working, some-one came in covered in lice. You could see them crawling in his hair. We could have just given him the lotion and told him to wash his hair, but I put on an apron and gloves, and stood behind him – where you stand is important – and he let me rinse the stuff through his hair. It took half an hour and as I worked, we could talk. Physical touch can release openness; it was a way for him to talk about what was worrying him.'

In May 2018 the journalist George Monbiot wrote a moving column in the *Guardian* about his experience of surgery for prostate cancer: 'The first revelation was the astonishing power of human kindness. The team that treated me, at the Churchill hospital in Oxford, made me feel I was part, however briefly, of a vast but close family. The consideration of the doctors and nurses, who managed to create the impression that they had all the time in the world, even as they were rushed off their feet; the instant responses of the ward and the triage team whenever I ran into trouble after I was discharged; the regular phone calls the surgeon made to see how I was coping: this was more than just professionalism. It felt like care in every sense. I am convinced that this attention was crucial to my recovery.'

Nursing care is powerful for both recipient and giver. Whitman described his experience in the Washington hospitals as 'the centre, circumference and umbilicus of my whole career', and, like many of the nurses quoted in this chapter, maintained that it had brought him to a deeper understanding of himself and his shared humanity. It is this precious and powerful insight that seems beleaguered.

(iv)

compassion

compassion, noun – Pity inclining one to help or be merciful, from Latin *pati pass*, to suffer.

The word is steeped in a long religious history, but has made a surprise comeback in healthcare policy documents in recent years. In a common statement of purpose, *Hard Truths*, in the aftermath of the public inquiry into the ill treatment of patients at Stafford Hospital run by the Mid Staffordshire NHS Foundation Trust, fifteen senior officials in the NHS and Department of Health declared: 'We ensure that compassion is central to the care we provide and respond with humanity and kindness to each person's pain, distress, anxiety or need. We search for the things we can do, however small, to give comfort and relieve suffering. We find time for patients, their families and carers, as well as those we work alongside. We do not wait to be asked, because we care.'

Compassion comes from the same Latin word as 'patient' – *pati*, meaning to suffer, so 'com-passion' literally means to suffer with someone. But it is not just about sharing an experience; ethical action is required and resilience is needed to avoid being overwhelmed by emotion. Each religious tradition has its own interpretation of the central role of compassion. In all three of the Abrahamic faiths, compassion is a central attribute of God. The word is mentioned as a name of Allah in all but one of the 114 verses of the Quran. Compassion is considered one of the three distinguishing marks of being a Jew. In the Chinese Buddhist tradition, compassion is expressed in the form of Kuan Yin, with her arms and eyes open; her name means 'one who listens to the sounds of the universe'. In the Tibetan Buddhist tradition, Avalokiteśvara has a thousand eyes to see suffering and a thousand arms to reach out to help. Buddhism suggests that the first requirement of compassion is not to turn away, often the instinctive response to suffering. Compassion is one of four qualities which support and reinforce each other, along with joy, equanimity and open-minded acceptance. Without joy and equanimity, compassion can lead to exhaustion.

Compassion can easily be marginalized in institutions, suggests researcher Dr Paquita de Zuleta. Drawing on evolutionary psychology and affective neuroscience, she argues that compassion is inhibited in competitive or threatening environments. She points out that human beings have three emotion systems: the first detects and responds to threat and is associated with fear, anxiety, anger and disgust; the second is linked to feelings of achievement, excitement and pleasure; and the third is the soothing system linked to feelings of contentment, safeness, serenity, connection – and essential to the expression of compassion. All three should be in balance and are appropriate in different circumstances. The danger is that the first restricts the soothing system. Much care work inevitably entails levels of anxiety, and when further pressure is added, such as targets for waiting times or bed throughput, fear can swamp the capacity for compassion. It may be an innate human capability, argues de Zuleta, but it is fragile. She warns that industrialized, marketized healthcare prioritises transactional care with measurable outcomes, and that squeezes out compassion. On a more positive note, she adds, it is inherently reciprocal, and is easy to recognize. It is also infectious – if you experience it, you are more likely to show it to another.

5

Three Hundred Decisions a Day

IN THE SURGERY

'It's such a little thing to weep –
So short a thing to sigh –
And yet – by Trades – the size of these
We men and women die!'

EMILY DICKINSON, 'It's such a little thing to weep',
Poems, 1896

The stark waiting room was quiet, the receptionists spoke in low voices on the phone, and the patients sat on the benches waiting, mostly in silence. When a door opened and a patient left the room, occasionally the doctor could be heard saying goodbye – the only voice to break the hush. As the doctor ushered each new patient into the consultation room, they carefully ensured they had shut the door. The routine nature of what I was observing obscured its extraordinary character: this is the only place where someone can ask a highly trained professional to listen, and be confident that whatever is said will be treated with confidence, respect, and without judgement. No money changes hands. This is an encounter grounded in the values of the welfare state: free at the point of need.

Every working day, nearly a million patients in the UK sit in similar waiting rooms to see a general practitioner. This form of medicine has been critical to the success of the NHS: within days of its launch in 1948, queues formed to sign up with GPs for the miracle of free medical care. It has saved countless lives and, critically, general practice ensured the astonishing political experiment of the NHS was affordable. GPs were given the role of deciding whether someone needed to see a hospital specialist, and became gatekeepers, managing and limiting the demand on expensive hospital services. Unlike in other healthcare schemes across Europe, no one sees a specialist without a GP referral. Of those million daily appointments, only 10 per cent will need a referral. Without the work of those general practitioners, this mass of ailments and suffering would swamp the system.

The GP's task is demanding: she has to identify and meet the needs of the people on the benches in the waiting room, but also to ensure that other parts of the health service are not overloaded with unnecessary investigations and referrals. Both of these requirements have intensified in recent decades as patient demands have increased and resources have been constrained. GPs are pivotal in managing the inherent tension between demand and an affordable supply of healthcare, and, as a result, are subject to intense political and social pressure. At the heart of this conundrum is the issue of care.

With the rise of scientific medicine, a perception gained ground that 'doctors cured and nurses cared', but this was never meaningful in general practice, and is arguably false in all medicine. As I shadowed a busy inner-city general practice, I grasped that the *only* way to do the job is through the prism of care as a highly developed, self-aware set of behaviours and values, many of which are poorly understood by wider society, and even by the patients themselves. 'Practice' is entirely the right word to apply to the work, because during every appointment the doctor is using her knowledge to assess multiple risks and her constant companions are uncertainty and an awareness of her limitations. What guides her through this territory of huge responsibility is her understanding of how to provide care. And, as I had discovered in other contexts, this care has been ignored, undervalued or is directly threatened.

The result is that the job is increasingly difficult to do, and GPs are voting with their feet and leaving the profession. In May 2019, for the first time in fifty years, the number of GPs in the UK dropped, despite repeated government commitments to increase the total. This prompted widespread media coverage, because, as we have seen with other parts of the health service, demand is rising: the number of appointments is growing at around 5 per cent a year. An ageing demographic and the rise in chronic conditions put pressure on GPs; the only hope of containing the cost of this increasing need is to have a strong, effective GP system, yet the profession is gripped by a retention and recruitment crisis. Already in 2015, the British Medical Association warned of the largest shortfall ever in trainees, and in subsequent years, the figures have dropped again, while the number taking early retirement is growing. Research for the Nuffield Trust has found that the ratio of GPs per 100,000 of the population fell from sixty-five in 2014 to sixty in just four years. The shortfall is predicted to triple by 2023/4. Without GPs to staff them, practices are closing; in May 2019 a sharp increase in closures grabbed the headlines, and commentators pointed out that the rate had been accelerating since 2013, despite government initiatives to help. The danger is that, as demand increases and GPs find themselves under more strain, workloads become intolerable; one in five do more than fifty consultations a day, one in ten do a staggering sixty, twice the safe limit, while seeing thirty or forty patients is common, with up to forty hospital letters to read and action, and the working day regularly stretching to more than twelve or thirteen hours. The Royal College of General Practitioners describes the job as now 'undoable'. The *Guardian* commented in an editorial in May 2019 that, while hospital waiting times tend to make headlines, 'the crisis in general practice is the most serious threat now faced by the NHS'.

Underlying this retention and recruitment crisis is a persistent frustration amongst many GPs that they cannot do the job in the way they believe it needs to be done. In part this is due to an historic underinvestment in primary care, only slowly being remedied (the prestige of hospital services has grabbed the lion's share of funding), but equally important has been a series of changes in which care practices have been marginalized – either regarded as irrelevant or they are in open conflict with new priorities. Over the last forty years, the average general practice has changed from a single doctor to a team of several, assisted by nurses, other healthcare professionals, a manager and administrative staff. The extension of surgery hours to improve convenience has led to doctors doing shifts. The cost of these changes has been less continuity of care. Patients see the next available doctor rather than developing a long-term relation-ship. In addition, the development of technology placed a new emphasis on gathering and analysing data rather than communi-cating with the patient. Efforts to root out poor-quality practice led to the introduction of the Quality and Outcomes Framework in 2004, which ensures that at every appointment the doctor is prompted to collect routine data on the patient. Following the horrific crimes of Dr Harold Shipman, a GP convicted in 2000 of murdering fifteen patients (and suspected of killing another 250), scrutiny has increased. Doctors have to be revalidated every five years, and there has been an increase in complaints, many of which require considerable time to resolve. At any one time, there are around 75,000 complaints against GPs under investigation. The time available to attend to a patient and listen carefully has been squeezed on several fronts.

Many of the changes may have brought benefits, but they also betray a lack of understanding of what the GP's job entails, it is argued. Most of those who write about healthcare or develop policy are educated, well off and healthy; their experience of the GP usually amounts to little more than the occasional pre-scription for antibiotics. Policy expertise has been dominated by hospital specialists (such as Professor Lord Ara Darzi, a cardiac surgeon). The priority is perceived to be convenience and choice for patients and this takes pre-eminence in the design of services and in media coverage; for example the extension of surgery opening times. But in the average surgery, such well off and healthy patients are a minority. A significant number of those in the waiting room will never get an explanation for their aches and pains – no organic cause will ever be found; the proportion of patients with 'Medically Unexplained Symptoms' varies from 20 to 40 per cent. Meanwhile, the bulk of those making GP appoint-ments are the frail elderly, the mentally ill, those with chronic conditions, or people caught up in chaotic, fragmented lives of addiction and abuse. Poverty breeds illness, and illness breeds more illness, generating co-morbidity in contexts with few spare resources to ease the suffering. Above all else, the GP's waiting room represents a complex challenge of care.

As I searched around to gain a deeper insight – I have had the good fortune so far to fall in the category of needing little from my GP – one surgery invited me to shadow their work. They suggested I sat in on consultations, attended all practice meet-ings and interviewed staff. Their motive was a keen interest in an account of their labour of care; they wanted it recognized and better understood. They passionately believed in the value of their work. Yet they felt continually undermined, frustrated by policy debates and organizational leadership which demonstrated little insight into their work.

I'll call the practice Edgerly Hill. A busy urban practice, it served patients from a cluster of large housing estates in a major UK city. The area was changing, and cranes reared overhead on building sites with hoardings emblazoned with adverts for apartments at prices beyond the reach of many of the long-term residents. Traditionally a relatively deprived area, it had absorbed successive waves of migrants over the last forty years. Many brought a family narrative of fleeing from violent conflict, or escaping poverty to build a better future for their children. The result was a densely populated area thick with histories which spanned the world.

On this winter Monday morning in the consultation room, the first appointment was a young Eastern European mother who had brought her young son. She talked of his breathing problems, and was worried about the persistent damp in her flat. The doctor, Tom, listened to the boy's chest and checked his medication; beyond that, there was little he could do, but she thanked him profusely for his time. Next, a young professional wanted the referral letter that his private health insurance required so that he could see a consultant about a problem with his toe nail. An emergency phone call came through: a daughter was anxious that her mother could be having a stroke. Tom asked a series of careful questions, and concluded she probably wasn't. It transpired later that the patient needed the inhaler she had misplaced. During the appointments, Tom made a point of turning away from his screen to face the patient; only when they left the room did he type up the notes. Next up, a middle-aged woman worried she had lost her libido, followed by a young woman who was feeling low and wanted antidepressants.

The patients arriving in Tom's consultation room represented the varied lives of this diverse neighbourhood. Most of
the Edgerly Hill staff – doctors, managers and nurses – had an
unusual degree of knowledge drawn from working here over
many years, intimately knowing families over several generations, through pregnancies, deaths, births, car accidents and
depressions. They had seen the children grow up and produce
children of their own; they had seen the parents sicken and
die. When the doctors gathered for their team meetings, they
helped each other piece together stories which spanned multiple
lives and ages, each chipping in with elements critical to the
overall picture, as they checked and rechecked diagnoses and
treatments.

Each of Tom's consultations rests on what the doctor and
philosopher Raymond Tallis describes as medicine's 'fathomless aquifers of implicit knowledge, understanding, custom
and practice'. (His choice of metaphor is a reminder of how, so
often, care is concealed.) One aspect of this is political; the GP
surgery has carried the standard, in a way no other organization
or profession has done, for the post-war welfare state's ideals
of equality, fraternity and solidarity. In the consultation room
Tom is expected to provide care for each patient with the same
degree of attention, be they a well-paid lawyer or a murderer,
someone suffering from terminal cancer or a person worried
about hair loss; and the last patient of the day is entitled to the
same quality of attention as the first.

This is the first characteristic of care: the patient's access to
the undivided attention of a highly trained professional. The
patient can reveal anything, and the doctor listens to what is
often a tangled account of anxiety, fear, pain, or even shame.
This listening is the most important part of the job, Tom
believes. It has been estimated that 85 per cent of the evidence
used to reach a diagnosis is derived from what the patient says,

with physical examinations adding only 7 per cent and diagnostic tests another 7 per cent. As the GP and blogger Jonathan Tomlinson writes, 'even in this highly technical age, by far and away the most powerful diagnostic tool a doctor has is their ability to listen. We elicit, understand and interpret our patients' stories, gain their trust and in so doing allow them to reveal their ideas, fears and expectations.'

The listening is no easy task: Tom has also to communicate he is listening with physical gestures, expressions of concern and encouragement. He has to give the patient confidence so that they can mention even details they may not regard as significant. Tom then sifts through the patient's detailed account to identify a correlation with his medical knowledge. There is always a danger of patient and doctor talking past each other, as one has the subjective experience, the other the medical; a doctor's role is akin to that of interpreter. Often, the task is one simply of reassurance, and the significance of that is all too easy to underestimate.

This complex task is expected to be completed within the allotted ten minutes. A considerable improvement on the two-minute appointment standard in the 1950s, it lags well behind consultation times in many other European countries. In Sweden the average is nearly twenty-three minutes. Such a short time belies the complexity of expectation, response, roles and performances, and yet most doctors still manage to accomplish the task; according to an NHS survey, 87 per cent of patients said the GP gave them enough time. Inevitably, that is often at the cost of the GPs' working longer hours, and in Edgerly Hill doctors routinely went well over the ten minutes with elderly patients who were managing complex regimes of medication.

The second characteristic of care, the GPs at Edgerly Hill insisted, was continuity. The relationships with patients built up over years generated patient trust, and, crucially, helped the

doctor to make the necessary clinical judgements about the
risks inherent in every appointment. An extraordinarily high
and sustained rate of major decision-making is required every
day, as the sociological research on general practice has always
pointed out: decisions affecting individual lives – and deaths –
the functioning of the NHS, and its costs. Alex, another doctor
at Edgerly Hill, calculated he made about 300 significant decisions a day. By the time he got home, he added, he would tell
his wife that he had no idea what they should eat for dinner:
he was incapable of making another decision. Only with deep,
sustained knowledge of the patient over a period of years could
such a volume of decisions be made accurately and swiftly,
argued the Edgerly Hill doctors. Continuity was essential to do
the job.

Helping them bear the burden of that responsibility was a
routine embedded in the Edgerly Hill practice but which has
been squeezed out in many other surgeries for lack of time: at
the end of every session, the doctors ran over summaries of each
appointment with a colleague or two, pooling their collective
experience, and checking the diagnosis. From their geographical knowledge of the surrounding streets and their biographical
knowledge of the families who lived in them emerged an understanding of care as not just maintaining an individual's health,
but something less tangible and much bigger: sustaining social
stability through a persistent containment of the suffering and
tragedies that destabilize lives, families and communities.

Tom's job required a particular kind of emotional stamina,
which can tolerate the misery, even despair, and hold the weight
of responsibility. Patients often changed as they entered the
consultation room, shedding their relatively confident public
persona, shifting into a more vulnerable version of themselves.
Their accounts offered glimpses of complex lives, like compelling film trailers, and for many of those suffering from poverty

and cultural dislocation, the possibility of relief for their ailments was remote. Managing that disappointment and maintaining trust in the relationship was part of Tom's achievement. Iona Heath, a former president of the Royal College of General Practitioners, described the GP's consultation room as the interface 'where the vast, undifferentiated mass of human distress and suffering meets the theoretical structures of scientific medicine and social sciences which have been developed to enable humanity, to a still very limited extent, to understand and control the experience of illness ... The doctor's role is to acknowledge and witness the suffering brought by illness.'

The patients offered a cornucopia of sensation – hot burning flashes, lumps on the leg, pains on the top of the head – along with a medley of anecdote and information. Some ailments might clear up on their own, others become life-threatening. The doctor has to keep in view both possibilities, but patients are unwilling to tolerate such uncertainty. A belief has grown that 'all truths about disease will ultimately reveal themselves', suggests E. J. Cassell in *The Nature of Suffering and the Goals of Medicine*; 'because of burgeoning technology, doctors and patients are behaving as though diagnoses can be known with certainty ... Many of the problems of current medicine, from high cost to depersonalization and overuse of technology, are methods of denying the inevitability of uncertainty. The hallmark of a clinician is their ability to tolerate uncertainty.' The GP and author Julian Tudor Hart argues that medicine can 'never achieve the virtual certainty possible in air travel or engine design' and admitted that 'right up to my last week in practice, I still feared making potentially serious mistakes, and with good reason. Any attempt to apply knowledge from human biology to specific real lives entails a significant margin of error.' As Alex, at Edgerly Hill, explained it to me: 'What strikes the fear of god into a GP is a patient coming in and saying, "I want this sorted." I might want to be six foot tall with a full head of hair, but it's not going to happen.' Failure of various kinds is an inevitable part of the job description, Alex continued. People die. Chronic conditions can cause years of suffering, and some pain has no medical explanation. A GP has to juggle the hope of the patient, the high expectations of society, and the limits inherent in their skill. They are trained to regard all their judgements as provisional and available for reconsideration if new relevant information emerges. Time is a routine part of the diagnostic process to sort the trivial from the more serious: 'Let's wait and see,' or 'Come back if the pain doesn't go away.' Equally, time can suddenly, unexpectedly, become critical. Few professions have failure so very close to every fragile success.

In one appointment, a young woman, desperately anxious, asked Tom if he could guarantee her mother wouldn't have another stroke; the only possible answer was no. On the basis of this answer, she insisted her mother went into hospital immediately. Again, the only possible answer was no.

I accompanied Tom on an afternoon of home visits. We climbed the concrete steps of the shabby post-war blocks. Beyond the forbidding front doors and wrought-iron security gates, the elderly women we visited had created richly decorated homes in their small flats, shrines to family and memory. The colours were vibrant and the furniture covered with luxurious fabrics of satin and velvet. The windows were draped with net. Mirrors, glass and heavy gilt-framed photographs glinted in the lamplight. Havens from an alien world beyond the front door.

Alex described how many of the patients at Edgerly Hill suffered from what he called the 'Ulysses syndrome', a form of profound homesickness. Having left or been forced to leave their homes many decades ago, often because of violent conflict, they now found that their British-born offspring had grown up and moved away. The elderly parents were betwixt and between;

they had lost their home in young adulthood, and they had lost their children to a culture they barely understood. The syndrome was particularly acute for women whose lives may have been entirely circumscribed by home and family, and who had never learnt to speak English or even to find their way around the immediate neighbourhood. The heartache often manifested itself in Medically Unexplained Symptoms, Alex believed: aches and pains for which the doctors could offer little relief but which brought the patient back to the surgery month after month. Fifteen years ago, unexplained abdominal pains led to a pattern of hysterectomies and appendectomies; now these patients were often treated with antidepressants. But neither eased the sense of displacement, of being caught adrift in a world they did not recognize. In one appointment, when Alex wanted to test a patient's memory, he asked her to name a local street; she couldn't. She was utterly dependent on her husband and children to navigate the world.

'As a GP you have to like –' Alex pauses to correct himself – 'no, more than like, you have to be interested in people. You need to be nosey. I'm drawn to the struggle of people whose lives are chaotic. Witnessing pain. It's so interesting, trying to connect with patients over time. I go on long journeys with them, sometimes over twenty years. A lot of the time people come wanting an explanation that fits, but you might not have one, or you might not be able to convince them of the one you have.'

Alex is short and wiry, full of a furious energy, with a quick-witted humour that ensures that in every practice meeting – no matter how dire the subject matter – he has everyone laughing. He flings his arms out to underline a point, and jumps to his feet to emphasize a question. These sudden, unpredictable movements make him fascinating to watch at work. His style of consultation is idiosyncratic; the briskness alternates with an intense curiosity in everyone who walks through his door. He fires off questions seemingly at random, gathering details of peoples' lives while taking their blood pressure, or listening to their chest: 'Where were you born? . . . What do you do?'

Alex's manner is akin to that of a chat-show host, yet bears the authenticity of his own character. 'There is a theatricality about me. My patients know that and they are part of it too. They play themselves. The performance is not superficial. I've grown into the persona I play and am comfortable with it. It's authentic and hard won. I've worked hard for many years and that has knocked off many edges. During that time, I've made mistakes. I've had to apologize to patients, and that can be really brutal. People have died sooner than they should have done. I know what it is like to be put through the wringer. There is always a process of reflective self-evaluation. That's why we do our feedback meetings in the practice; my colleagues scrutinize my work and I have nowhere to hide. That's very exposing. But in medicine, the margin of error is always very large.

'I feel that I am at my most genuine with patients. There is no game play. That is most apparent in end-of-life care. That interests me a lot. At that stage, someone is not playing any more games; they've not got time.

'There can be very powerful, startling moments in this job. I had one patient who was an alcoholic epileptic, and I used to visit him in his flat. It was completely bare, apart from a mattress on the carpeted floor, and he was incontinent and vomiting a lot. When I opened the door, flies swarmed out. But he was charming and funny, and his humanity shone through, even while my shoes were sticking to the carpet. You can find humanity bursting through everywhere, and part of my job is to try to respond to it.'

When colleagues are reviewing cases, Alex's mind works like a form of radar, scanning his memory to find connections in the many-layered social terrain of the nearby streets. He makes frequent interjections: 'She's the one with the mother who has a heart condition ... Isn't he the one whose son had a kidney problem? ... Her daughter died ten years ago.'

He started out wanting to be an architect, and it was not until his mid-twenties that he changed tack. 'Architects are driven by a sense of order and a desire to control environments. I grew up in a very disordered environment, with an alcoholic father, and I went to boarding school, a brutal place. I was an ex-pat child. As a result, I was very scared of people and their unpredictability, until I met my partner, who is the essence of calm and order. Then I decided that I liked people more than buildings. I changed career.

'My upbringing left me with a real interest in outsiders and injustice. I love working in a diverse area like this, and the occasional chaos. We try to find ways through it; we are sorting problems out all the time – or trying to. I like lots of plates spinning at the same time.'

Alex admits he likes the relentless pace of a GP practice, and it is no accident that he is a long-distance runner.

'We serve a few thousand people in a very small area. It's parochial, but we have an impact. We are witnessing these lives. Sometimes we are clever and we get the diagnosis spot on, but other times not. I call it the pendulum of medicine, and it keeps swinging – one day you get it right, the next you miss something. A great chunk of humility is needed. If someone escapes an abusive relationship or recovers from depression, that's great. I'm trying to help people steer their way through. Our great privilege is that we ask questions. We come across all kinds. One patient had assaulted his wife, but then he had been assaulted in Iraq by Saddam Hussein's police. People are never one thing: we are so much worse than our best act, and so much better than our worst one.

'As doctors, we are quite defended and our training helps us. That's how we can cope. Humour is a big way of getting through – recognizing the sheer absurdity of life. That's the glory of it.

'The NHS is a political football. I've seen the political short-termism, I've seen the wheel come right round again. We are watched as GPs, but I have my own approach to the churn of reform. Stay in the herd – we're wildebeest on migration. Don't fall behind or you get picked off; don't lunge for the green grass. Stick in the middle, mill and moo. Mill and moo!'

These days, he sees a new threat: a type of patient who uses private healthcare and expects investigation procedures that he regards as a waste of money and time. 'Young entitled professionals come in demanding this and that, and they take up more time than they should. But they will get old, and when they get their first proper illness, such as cancer, or their child is sick, then let's talk turkey. Then we all know where we are.'

Alex has a vivid understanding of how successful lives can suddenly become precarious, because he deals every day with multiple forms of vulnerability and dependence, and this, he asserts, is the reality of human lives, not those few decades of youth and privilege which a few enjoy.

'The heaviest use of the NHS is by the elderly and the very young. Most healthy middle-aged people – and they are the ones who make the decisions about the NHS – have had little need of it yet. They focus on issues such as seven-day working for doctors, which is irrelevant for most of my patients.'

'Will family doctors be replaced by artificial intelligence?' I ask.

Alex is unruffled. 'It can't, because we are social animals, and we need relationships.' He pauses, thoughtful. 'Perhaps those who don't have money will end up with computers.

'I don't get overwhelmed by the suffering I see, but by the decisions I have to make. Hundreds a day, and I have to make them very quickly. I've never had a dull day, ever. Every day, I think, this is interesting. My job just gets better every year, because you know more about these families and their lives. It gets richer.'

In *A Fortunate Man*, his influential study of a rural doctor in the 1960s, John Berger asked, 'What is the effect of facing, trying to understand, hoping to overcome the extreme anguish of other persons five or six times a week? ... the anguish of dying, of loss, of fear, of loneliness, of being desperately beside oneself, the sense of futility.' Alex and Tom were encountering such anguish five or six times a day. Human suffering in many different forms washed through each surgery as regular as the tide. The doctors had the task of Sisyphus, who, in the classical myth, rolled the huge stone up the mountain every day, only for it to roll back down.

A weeping new mother explained how she was living in a tiny flat, and was exhausted by trying to keep her two children from disturbing her sick parents; her father was forced to sleep on the sitting-room floor. An elderly Turkish woman, shaking with fear as tears rolled down her cheeks, explained in broken English how she had been deemed fit to work and was being switched to Job Seeker's Allowance. She would have to attend a job centre daily to apply online for jobs that she knew she would not get.

The Edgerly Hill doctors encountered in their patients the sense of futility Berger described, and struggled to offer meaning – a diagnosis – for their suffering. It was hard to witness, and I shifted uneasily in the background. The doctors knew that often their efforts were limited. Even when a patient reported feeling better, the queue outside the door remained, as people sat anxiously waiting for their ten-minute slot. There was never enough time.

'We do not understand how to take the measure of a doctor. What he is doing ... when he is no more and no less than easing – and occasionally saving – the lives of a few thousand contemporaries,' writes Berger.

Many of the patients at this surgery have been written off as failures and misfits by a judgemental society. If you can do little or no work, in what way does your life have a value to society? Where do you find respect and recognition? The doctor's appointment was a critical moment of attention from someone with authority and power, offering, at its best, recognition of the individual's unique history, and thus becoming a vital prop to help make sense of chaotic lives.

'Any general culture acts as a mirror which enables the individual to recognize himself/herself – or at least those parts of himself [sic] which are socially permissible. The culturally deprived have far fewer ways of recognizing themselves. A great deal of their experience – especially the emotional and introspective – has to remain unnamed . . . the doctor represents their lost possibility of understanding and relating to the outside world,' writes Berger. He described the role of the general practitioner as a 'clerk of records'. More important even than their uncertain, limited role of healing, they served as witness, expressing a vital practice of solidarity.

The review meetings at the end of every surgery demonstrated that Berger's insight into the GP as a clerk of records is as true today as fifty years ago. A giddy tour of dozens of lives in the space of fifteen minutes, in which the heart attack of one patient could be related perhaps to the problems of his sister, and the death of his father, fifteen years before; it was a mapping of the neighbourhood in bodies and their travails. In most city neighbourhoods, lives have become anonymous and memory has been privatized, but here, in this practice, was a plotting of lives in these streets. On occasions, it became freighted with tragedy: the prison sentence, a parent's suicide, the sibling's self-harm, prostitution, rape and child sex abuse.

At a conference, a GP admitted to me that care was the difficult part of his job, and he found the 'giving of self' draining, but
he also knew that it could be the most important. He described
his role as one of reframing his patients' expectations. 'They
told me stories,' he said, and he had to subtly change them. As
at Edgerly Hill, his practice had kept up the routine of a midday
meeting to discuss cases, and he believed this was essential.
'Speaking out loud is powerful. It is different from thinking
something in your head, different physiologically, because you
use other parts of the brain to generate and perform speech. It's
like in Ursula Le Guin's Earthsea trilogy of novels, in which
the central conceit is that you have to know or learn the name
of something in order to unlock the power of that thing. The
naming brings a magical power.'

It was not yet 10 a.m. and Liz, level, dogged and cheerful,
another of the partners at Edgerly Hill, had already had to
deal with a woman who insisted that 'her eyes were gone with
crying'; a young boy who energetically yelped that 'it burned'
when she touched his abdomen; and a young woman with a
pain in her tummy when she laughed. The boy's case was
puzzling. He seemed a normal, lively boy, but he kept coming
back to the surgery. The young woman had a history of self-
harm. None of these cases had a clear diagnosis. Much of the
time Liz was providing reassurance. Anxiety is the currency of
every GP practice.

The young woman apologized profusely for taking up Liz's
time. 'I shouldn't have come – it's probably nothing,' she said,
before admitting, 'Even a five minute chat on the phone with
you helps.'

How can one explain the value of the doctor's role in containing fragility just by being a stable, continuous presence in
someone's life? It may only be ten minutes once a month, but

it's a moment of commitment and reliability in lives which may not have much of either.

'I have poison in my face,' a patient declared, 'pins and needles down the side of my body like fire, but livelier.' Another announced, 'I feel weak in my hands.' Yet another offered symptoms: 'I feel a pulse all over. I crave sweet things.' Liz's job is part interpreter, part educator as she tries to establish a shared language about pain and illness. A task made all the harder by the fact that she and the patient might not share a language, and are dependent on interpreters. Many brought their own cultural understandings of health and the role of doctors; one Ukrainian woman asked if her blood pressure was related to the cycles of the moon. Assured it did not, she did not look convinced. Trust in a doctor is a cultural construct, depending on a set of long histories – of science, the medical profession, the NHS – combined with biographical experience.

Next in was an elderly couple. She had just been discharged from hospital. Her husband was carrying a large bag of her medications, but the hospital had confused them with warnings of blood clots, and there had been a muddle about which prescription to pick up from where. It took fifteen minutes to disentangle and explain, and the patient left with prescriptions the thickness of a paperback book. They were full of apologies for taking up Liz's time.

Then a woman asking for contraception because she is going 'home', and, she whispered, 'No does not mean no.' Liz nodded her understanding.

'I see so much pain – but also a desperate hope,' she told me later. 'As an experienced GP, I have become reconciled to the fact that simply being there is something which is worth doing. Sometimes "we are the treatment", and you have to accept that your role is not to change people. You try and find every person interesting. It is as if each person is a ball of wool – you follow the thread until you find a bit of humanity. That is care. You need distance, but you also need empathy. You feel their pain, but you don't suffer it. You can't take it on.

'We have so many roles. There is the obvious role of diagnosing treatable illness; we listen to a story, and arrive at a working diagnosis. Hopefully, we are helping people to live healthier lives by managing their illness. But we also have other roles, and reassurance is a big part of our job. It is important when we say, "You don't have an illness, and you don't need to worry." We can offer more reassurance by saying, "It was a good reason to come, but now, don't worry." People don't recognize the value of that.

'We are an accessible part of the establishment. People can reach us, unlike the bank manager or the MP or perhaps their boss. That's incredible, and sometimes I think that's our main role; we listen to people and we are their advocate.'

Later, when we are sitting in the staff room surrounded by coffee mugs and boxes of biscuits donated by grateful patients, I ask her to define care. She pauses before she speaks.

'It is the most important thing. People going through tough times, or who are in the final stage of their lives, and need to feel cared for. It is completely different to the way you care for people you love, because it's not based on an emotional bond. As GPs, we are quite controlling, and care is partly about control and order. Our work definitely requires empathy, and it is also about curiosity in people's stories. I really *like* people; they are remarkable. Everyone has something to offer, and you learn so many things. I want to know what makes people tick.

'Feeling that you may have helped someone is very rewarding. You get lovely letters, and presents, but you don't need to have that kind of appreciation to feel that it was worthwhile. I know the benefit of what I'm doing.' She comes to a stop. Hesitantly, she picks up again: 'It feels exposing – a bit big-headed – to talk like this. I don't want to beat my drum, but it feels like a valuable job to do. I'm acutely aware of the human condition. We see things in a way that few other people do – all kinds of human experiences on a daily basis. Other people wouldn't believe it if they knew. I meet up with friends once a week for a drink, and the other women talk about their work, but I have to be very careful, for confidentiality reasons, and besides I don't want to gossip. We hear remarkable stories, but they shouldn't be used for the entertainment of friends. If I told them about my day, it would be too much for other people to process; they might not even believe me. No one else has this kind of perspective. I am exposed to the extremes of life and it changes you. I enjoy that, and the more so as I go on. It has made me a better person. I'm much more tolerant than I would have been if I hadn't done this job. The job has made me humble.

'Life is very challenging for many people, and yet there is immense humanity in people who have experienced terrible things and still have a positive attitude; people with learning difficulties who have a lot to offer; people with no education but with a lot of emotional intelligence. I recognize that people have value even though they may not appear that way.'

Liz saw patients for four and half hours without time to even sip a cup of tea, let alone make one. Practical, down-to-earth and capable, she had extraordinary emotional and physical stamina. She also had a clarity about her job, her ability to do it and its value: these three are rare achievements in a working life. She had in abundance what the literary critic Kate Kellaway describes as 'the luxury of being useful'. With that came self-respect, and a stability of self; she knew where she stood in the world and why.

Above her desk, she had covered the noticeboard with photos of her busy family life over almost two decades. Babies, teenagers, damp walks, seaside trips. 'Patients like them – they say it makes me human. There's a balance between self-disclosure and holding back. Nothing must detract from the most important person in the consultation: the patient. I spend too much time in this room; it was eleven hours on Monday, over ten yesterday and it will be twelve hours today. These photos remind me of my other world – that of home and family – and it *is* two worlds.'

Over half of the appointments at this surgery are related in one way or another to mental health: depression, anxiety or a specific diagnosis such as psychosis.

'The best we can sometimes offer,' says Tom, 'is a containing, witnessing sort of presence. Over a long period, I can feel I've made a difference.'

Above his desk in his consultation room, he has hung an abstract art print of geometric shapes. It reflects Tom's precise restraint and the emotion underlying it. His room is meticulously tidy, and his manner exemplifies the ordering imperative of his work. He greets each patient with a handshake, and is thorough in his questioning, frequently overrunning the allotted time. To Alex's chat-show host, he would be the vicar with his polite but gentle formality. He explains why he feels Edgerly Hill's way of working is under siege.

'We are very proud and committed to our model of care and feel it is not well understood. The focus is on what can be measured, such as data collection and targets. No one has found a way fully to measure continuity of care or its value, but we know it reduces hospital admissions. How do you work out the value of the central doctor-patient relationship and how it plays out over time? We get paid, praised and exhorted to offer convenience, access, and choice. But, by definition, access is not compatible with continuity of care.

'There are also dangers in the current emphasis on evidence-based medicine. We know that the process is skewed by the pharmaceutical industry, which can fund research; the negative findings are repressed, and there is a publication bias. The principles of evidence-based medicine play into the idea that healthcare can be done by algorithm and that it is just a matter of collating enough data. At present, the National Institute of Clinical Excellence (NICE) insists on the importance of clinical judgement, but for how much longer? Society might decide that a family doctor is a luxury that can no longer be afforded.

'A lot of what we deal with is the result of poverty – addiction, obesity, lung disease. We live in a deeply unequal society, in which the physical and mental health of the poor and marginalized suffers. As GPs, we see the extraordinary circumstances of adversity that some people have to cope with. I know we're working to put a sticking plaster on a broken system, but that's not futile. Of course I question the benefit and the impact of my work. The current paradigm in healthcare is discovering risk factors in well people and treating them. So, for example, you can have high blood pressure, have no symptoms, and yet be on several medications. It is based on good epidemiology, but for individuals it makes no sense – it is based on population-wide interventions. What we do medically is open to challenge as to its effectiveness, but what is genuinely valuable, I believe, is the interpersonal relationship.

'Touch is a powerful form of communication, I'm aware of that. It's part of the theatre of the consultation room. The psychoanalyst and thinker Michael Balint talked of the "drug doctor", and by that he meant the power of the relationship itself. If I seem bored, indifferent or hurried, the consultation will be less therapeutic. We have a social role and people have expectations of the encounter with the doctor. If I didn't feel the patient's pain, I wouldn't be authentic. Alongside the performance of the role, you have to be authentic to yourself; that means GPs do their job in very different ways.

'The concept of the "wounded healer" is important – the

person who has themselves been hurt or damaged has deeper insight into the processes of healing. As a doctor, you choose to spend your life intimately involved in other people's distress. At some level, it meets your own needs. A big part of what keeps me engaged is emotional identification: trying to develop an understanding of what it is to be in the patient's position. I'm good at keeping boundaries, but there is pain that goes along with that. It's striking that Dr Sassall, the doctor portrayed by Berger in *A Fortunate Man*, committed suicide. And a doctor who wrote about his work in the East End of London in the 1980s, David Widgery, died of a suspected overdose. We deal with a great deal of pain on a daily basis, and there can be a personal cost. There is a deep sense of connection with the patient at that level of vulnerability and intimacy. But you gain an amazing understanding of how people live. It's a privilege to have this in-depth view of society, which most people don't ever see.

'Work can leave me frazzled: a combination of the level of emotional engagement, the volume of decisions required, and the quantity of personal encounters. That's why none of us works more than four days a week. We work less than our predecessors. The old-style GP probably did nine surgeries a week, but the work has intensified – we have more information at our fingertips to review, there are more investigations to coordinate and results to collate. You have to integrate all these disparate pieces of information from different time points into a diagnosis.

'It's a very humbling job, but the shadow side of that is a sense of inadequacy that can flip into arrogance. That is very dangerous in a doctor. The job feels useful, but often your role is very limited. We get things wrong on a regular basis.'

A young man comes in complaining of a cold and, like many, asks for antibiotics. Tom explains that they would do nothing for a virus, and as he is talking, he observes the young man, who is on anti-psychotic drugs. Tom asks if he is taking his medication, and he insists that he is, and that he just has a cold. Tom persists, as skilful as a fly fisherman. Finally, a story tumbles out: there's a girl at his church, there have been accusations that he has been harassing her, he wants to be in hospital. He wants to be back under the supervision of the community mental-health treatment team. No one will ever know what crisis has been narrowly averted in that precious fifteen minutes.

There is a gravity to Tom's manner. He reassures a student worried about feeling low that she has done the right thing in coming to see him. He pays his patients the respect of taking each of them seriously. Every time he does so, he contributes to the trust people put in his profession; doctors come a close second to nurses in ratings for trust, both scoring over 90 per cent.

A vicar is charged with the 'cure' of souls, but the definition of 'cure' is close to 'care' – emotional and spiritual support and guidance. The vicar, like the GP, has a role circumscribed by geography, with clearly demarcated boundaries. There are similar expectations of access, attention and compassion. They are both in the business of offering reassurance to the anxious. They bear witness to suffering and offer the small comforts of solidarity and respect. Both can offer some degree of affirmation of the person, and of their dignity. But they have always had different questions to answer. The question to the vicar is, 'Why? And why me?' The question to the doctor is, 'What is wrong with me?' The decline of faith leaves the first questions unanswerable, even unaskable. Perhaps that loads the other question with the full burden of anxiety, and the doctor has to fill the vacuum left by the priest. They may be expected to take on the task of making sense of the suffering – and that is sometimes beyond their skill.

*

On a home visit with Tom, we visited a man who was bed-bound, and cared for erratically by two sons, both with experience of the criminal justice system. The sons also had the care of a third brother with profound mental-health problems. Local-authority carers came into the small flat twice a day. On our visit, one of the sons described how his brother had got into a rage, smashing furniture and crockery. The curtains were closed, even though it was the middle of the day. Tom did what he could to reassure and check on medication. We moved on to the next visit, to a man who had received a diagnosis of terminal cancer. He had just moved into his girlfriend's flat, and he sat amongst the boxes, stoical and calm, as he discussed how he wanted to be cared for at the end of his life. He told Tom that he wanted to go into a hospice to die, but acknowledged that he had not yet dared tell his girlfriend.

Back at the surgery, a woman in her mid-seventies had come in for a sick note. She had been off work for a few weeks and needed to get back. Given that she was well past retirement age, the doctor was curious.

'Yes, I love my work as a cleaning supervisor,' she laughed, explaining her job enthusiastically, and then her cheerfulness faltered. Her husband was sick and had been for a check-up at the hospital. 'They talked of "a year",' she said, suddenly looking uncertain and afraid. Then she added quietly, 'But what can you expect at this stage?' Her calm question exposed a remarkable soul. The following week, I heard in a meeting that a routine blood test had indicated that she also had cancer.

In the course of the two weeks I shadowed the practice, I saw a model of care which has been at the centre of a bitter debate over the last thirty years. Three long-term trends have combined to challenge many of the principles Alex, Liz and Tom hold dear and to leave them operating in a system often uncomprehending of the value of their work.

The first has been a change of policy as a succession of
governments since the 1980s has introduced market mechanisms into general practice to improve efficiency and financial
accountability. The result has been a series of reorganizations
of the relationship between GPs and the rest of the NHS, each
time requiring huge adaptation. Competition, it was believed,
would drive up standards and reduce costs. To ensure the
market could operate effectively, it was necessary to break
down healthcare services (investigations, procedures and prescriptions) and health (biological results such as blood pressure
and cholesterol) and illness (diabetes or cancer) into units that
were measurable. Once there was measurable data, prices for
an internal NHS market and targets could be set. The Quality
and Outcomes Framework introduced in 2004 laid down a raft
of measures against which the work of GPs would be assessed,
with funding tied to implementation. Part of the rationale was to
weed out poor practice. But it also hugely increased the amount
of administration and brought bitter complaints that many
important aspects of GPs' work could not be measured and
were consequently disregarded. Data collection took a central
place in the job, with a new emphasis on how technology could
increase efficiency. At the same time, evidence-based medicine
has increasingly been codified and incorporated into 'decision-
support software', which urges doctors to use templates to make
clinical decisions. 'Medicine is changing from a craft concerned
with the uniqueness of each encounter to a mass manufacturing
industry. Doctors are becoming proletarians not artisans,' concludes the academic Steve Iliffe.

General practice was being industrialized, argued the critics, as a new focus emerged on population-wide preventative
health, such as tracking and medicating large numbers for
blood pressure. Incentives, targets, data collection and dead-
lines for specific interventions – for example smoking cessation

or flu jabs – were linked to funding. One of the nurses at Edgerly Hill commented to me after one appointment to give a patient an injection that he 'had just made £28 for the practice'. When I mentioned the remark to Tom, he admitted he was disappointed; their practice tried hard to keep this kind of transactional commercialism at bay. They tried to maintain what amounted to a Chinese wall between the management's handling of this bureaucracy and the clinical staff. In their defence, proponents of the reforms would argue that variations in the quality of general practice have been reduced. But the cost has been increased impersonalization for both doctor and patient. The doctor loses autonomy and, burdened with data collection, finds there is less space for listening and relationship; many GPs are so intent on their computer screens, they scarcely look at the patient. The patient is reduced to a set of numbers – age and statistics – to judge risk.

'Commercializing and industrializing processes are a confusing and destructive force [in healthcare]. They deflect, deform and ultimately demoralize staff motivation and imagination,' argues one of the most passionate critics, GP Julian Tudor Hart. The market is 'based on profit motivation: extreme division of labour; replacement of human labour with machines, and from that have come huge gains in productivity. But what has also happened is dehumanized labour.' None of this is appropriate or effective in healthcare, he warns, adding that 'media discussion and professionals deplore the dehumanization of care. It is not science which dehumanizes, but the market model.'

In a policy report the major healthcare think tank, the King's Fund, referred to general practice as a 'service industry' and lamented that it had 'lagged behind other service industries in achieving productivity gains from embracing technology'. Such a position leads to an agenda of meeting 'consumer' expectations of convenience and availability: seven-day working, and walk-in clinics. The consultation is reframed as a transaction, and patients are asked to fill in satisfaction questionnaires.

Policies based on the market model give little recognition to the burden of suffering Alex, Tom and Liz are dealing with, and how continuity makes their job possible. Only the strength of relationships built up over years sustains their capacity to maintain trust. But in a policy debate which demands quantitative evidence, their model of general practice has struggled to make its case: how do you measure the value of reassurance and relationship? Only recently has a study managed to demonstrate the effectiveness of continuity by showing that patients who saw different GPs were twice as likely to be admitted to hospital, but it is demoralizing that it takes a statistic to make the argument, not a doctor's professional experience.

The phrase 'patient choice' has been sprinkled liberally through political speeches and manifestos for several decades as a central aim of healthcare reforms. Perhaps voters find its repetition reassuring, but the philosopher and anthropologist Annemarie Mol argues that the 'logic of choice' is diametrically opposed to the 'logic of care', and cannot but compromise the latter. In her research in a diabetes clinic in the Netherlands, she explored the tension between the two. 'Good care is not a matter of making well-argued individual choices, but is something that grows out of collaborative and continuing attempts to attune knowledge and technologies to diseased bodies and complex lives,' she writes. As has been evident at Edgerly Hill, Mol believes that 'the ideal of good care is silently incorporated in practices and does not speak for itself . . . Given that it is under threat, it is time to put it into words.'

Choice is a deeply political concept, she argues, and across Western culture huge commercial and personal resources are invested in encouraging the desire for choice, selling those choices and persuading us how to make them. She suggests it is a 'disciplining technique,' a way of making people responsible for their fate. But in healthcare, no choice is straightforward, because it involves multiple uncertainties. The 'logics' of choice and of care are both needed at times, but the danger is that if choice is privileged, care is ignored, and at that point they come into conflict. 'Care is a process; it does not have clear boundaries. It is open-ended. It is a matter of time. Care is not a product that changes hands but a matter of various hands working together (over time) towards a result,' Mol writes.

Diabetes, the subject of her study, cannot be cured, so the goal has to be care not cure. Given the sharply rising incidence of diabetes and other chronic incurable conditions in Western countries, definitions of care are a central issue in the development of healthcare. The aim in diabetes, claims Mol, is to strike a balance between a long life and a happy one. 'What characterizes good care is a calm, persistent, but forgiving effort to improve the situation of the patient or to keep it from deteriorating.' The doctor doesn't present information so the patient can make a choice, but rather the two of them are collaborating, sharing different forms of knowledge and experience. There is no one-off moment when all the information is available to allow a choice to be made; diseases and bodies are too unpredictable for that. Instead care allows for such uncertainty by being vested in an ongoing relationship.

Mol's writing can be read as a careful elaboration and vigorous defence of the work of doctors like Alex, Liz and Tom. Her concluding pages are a powerful manifesto in which she argues that the logic of care should be applied to other areas of life, because it incorporates 'a raw honesty about failure and misery. Disease, death, suffering: care begins by facing these. They are not marginalized ... pseudo certainty is not invoked. Doubt does not preclude action. The attitude is experimental; you interact with the world while seeking what brings improvement and what does not. In the logic of care, actors do not have fixed tasks, [and] the action is more important than the actor.'

The model of care in general practice is a powerful but fragile construct, the outcome of decades of professional and institutional history, social consensus and cultural expectations. It is a far cry from its origins in the surgeon-apothecaries who, with their limited medical knowledge, were an option of last resort. The workload of a modern GP bears little relationship to that of their predecessors in the early twentieth century, who signed up to Lloyd's lists (named after Lloyd George, who brought in the first form of health insurance in 1911) and spent most of their time issuing sickness certificates so that patients could claim unemployment benefit. It is very different from the early days of the NHS, when general practice was chronically underfunded; the 1950 Colling Report found unheated waiting rooms, people queuing in the street, and consultation rooms with no couch and only one chair. GPs had been relegated to the bottom of the medical pecking order. They had to wait nearly twenty years after the founding of the NHS to be properly funded, with disgruntlement frequently reaching crisis point – mass resignations were threatened in 1957, and the early 1960s saw thousands of GPs emigrating to Australia, New Zealand and Canada for better pay and conditions. Only in the late 1960s was there a reinterpretation of the role, a new perspective on patients as unique and interesting individuals, and the fascination with 'narrative medicine' emerged. It was an expression of the intellectual optimism of the time, a deep faith in human capability, underpinned by a political commitment to human rights. As GP Margaret McCartney suggests, GPs took on a social role: 'being a businessman, missionary or socialist were the three reasons to become a GP, and in the 1970s you saw many more of the last emerging'. As that generation of GPs comes to the end of their working lives, the question is: which role will their successors opt for. The profession is deeply divided. Some have chosen the businessman, and work as salaried employees for the private companies which are taking over an increasing number of practices. Doctors lose their autonomy, and become subject to the organizational imperatives of a profit-seeking company.

In the nineteenth century, when a doctor had little medical skill, his job was a performance, colluding with the hopeful patient that he could help, and his main task was to ensure he was paid. What painfully and slowly evolved was a profession with the highest ethical standards and a deep humanitarian commitment. It has proved a remarkable achievement, but it is now squeezed from every side. 'There is a tension between the consumerist values of society,' suggests Raymond Tallis in his history of medicine, *Hippocratic Oaths*, 'and the values that have hitherto informed medicine at its best; values that drove it from a system beleaguered by fraud, venality and abuse of power to a genuinely caring profession.' There will always be healthcare for those who can pay for it, but the NHS represented an ideal of solidarity regardless of income. The risk is that we lose sight of Berger's conclusion in *The Fortunate Man*, as relevant today as it was in the Forest of Dean fifty years ago: 'Only when we understand how to value the life of an individual being, can we value the labour of a general practice doctor in the ways he sustains that life.'

(v)

pity

Pity, noun – Sorrow and compassion aroused by another's condition.

Pity, verb – Feel sorrow for the misfortunes of, take pity on – feel or act compassionately.

Perhaps it is in the nature of care, so prone to abuse and failure, to bankrupt the words used to describe it. That has proved the fate of pity. In all my research, no one ever used the word in an interview unless it was emphatically to reject it. Healthcare professionals regarded the word as toxic; it has been drilled out of them. Relationships of care are charged with unequal power, and pity has become contaminated by its history as a tool for patronizing condescension; it has too often tipped into the contempt which haunts care. Few words can be more loathed in the English language. Yet it has a grand history. *Pitie* was the word used by the French philosopher Jean Jacques Rousseau to describe the 'primitive instinct' of open-heartedness, which was too often sadly eroded by civilization. The individual's 'expansive heart cries with their pain, sighs with their suffering but the worldly man yearns for pre-eminence and his pitie withers under his ambition.'

The roots of the word 'pity' lie in the Latin for 'dutifulness', in the old French for 'compassion', and in the Middle English for 'mildness', 'clemency' or 'mercy'. All these magnificent associations have got lost in contemporary usage. Its close association with the Latin word *pietas* brings the whiff of hypocrisy. No one is supposed to feel pity or want to be pitied. The only acceptable use of the word is 'self-pity', and even that provokes distaste.

Yet we were once unabashed to admit our desire for pity. In *The Death of Ivan Ilyich*, Tolstoy writes: 'What most tormented Ivan Ilyich was that no one pitied him as he wished to be pitied. At certain moments after prolonged suffering he wished most of all (though he would be ashamed to confess it) for someone to pity him as a sick child is to be pitied.' Gwen Raverat Darwin recollects how in the late nineteenth century her grandfather, Charles Darwin, was always ill. She writes that, in her Victorian childhood, everyone else in the family imitated the much-loved grandfather and enjoyed being nursed by one family member or another: 'it was a distinction and a mournful pleasure to be ill . . . always delightful to be pitied and nursed'. When we are suffering, we are comforted by the concern of those caring for us, but we no longer admit, with Raverat's honesty, that experiencing pity from the right person can be 'delightful'.

Empathy has replaced pity. The shift reveals important changes in the understanding of care and what motivates it. The etymology of 'pity' tied together three ideas: duty, sorrow and mildness (best understood as gentleness). Duty is now regarded as a grim constraint on personal freedom, while mildness in this sense has been lost altogether, and clemency is rarely used. Instead the focus is on empathy as the motivation for care; with it comes the demanding expectation that the carer can share or at least imagine a set of emotions in the patient. I can't argue for pity's rehabilitation – there are times when words need to rest and recuperate – but it's worth remembering what we are losing.

6

Bearing Witness

'So we bear witness,
Despite ourselves, to what is beyond us.'

GEOFFREY HILL, 'Funeral Music',
New and Collected Poems, 1952–92

Sitting in an empty room of an office block on a Midlands industrial estate, my eye keeps coming back to two banners emblazoned with an elderly lady's face creased with smiles, some flowers and someone leaning over to help, their expression kindly. The home-care company I've come to visit makes a business from kindness. Down the corridor is an engineering and heating company; ironically, these neighbouring firms are both selling warmth.

Sue, one of the home-care workers, rarely comes to these offices; she is usually either visiting a client or sitting in her car between calls. Her contact with the company and her colleagues is by phone app; she clocks in for each visit and clocks out at the end; an alert goes off in the office if she is running late. The work is both closely supervised and yet lonely.

'I absolutely love my job, but I do have days when I don't know how I've survived,' Sue admits with a soft smile. She had little to say, she insisted at the start of the interview, but before long she is talking with barely a pause. 'One of my clients is very anxious and many of the carers refuse to go back. Her family is emotionally distant and they see the woman she was, rather than who she is now. I have a stomach ache every time I go in because I am so worried about what she'll be like – she can be screeching and everything might be all over the place, and it can be hard work to get her to calm down.' Sue pauses and reflects, 'You sort of need to be in control while letting her take the initiative. She needs to get a lot off her chest and you have to listen. I find ways to close down her anxiety. She's one of my hardest clients. There can be a constant stream of criticism and everything is wrong. That can be very challenging. She was a university lecturer, and she can't accept that she's old and needs help, but then she tells me stories, and she is so interesting and she reminds me of my nanny. I get nervous, but she's worth it.

'Another client is amazing because of her determination. She's quite eccentric. She is my last call of the day and that keeps me going. It's always a lovely call, even if she's been ill. She makes me smile and has a great sense of humour. She trusts us and asks our advice.

'One client has third-stage dementia. You're lucky if she will let you do any personal care. She can be aggressive and sometimes she can sit in a chair for three days without moving, and there will be faeces everywhere. She is clear and interesting one day, and the next she might be talking to her teddy bear. She's asked me to leave in the past. I got worried about her; everybody seemed prepared to let her slide. Once she went for days without

personal care and there was no food in the fridge. I reported it
and the dementia crisis team stepped in. It can be upsetting – I
think, it could be my family and another carer might not be as
caring as me.'

The company Sue works for is about as good as it gets in
home care: their minimum length of visit is an hour. She has a
chance to build up relationships with clients, which she finds satisfying, but the cost puts the company well beyond the budget
of local-authority services. It serves privately funded clients in
prosperous leafy suburbs. But even at this top end of the market,
Sue's skilful efforts with her clients receive meagre reward.

'I work around dropping the kids at school and picking them
up. I give them their tea, and then when my husband is home,
I go back to work. It can be very rushed – getting the kids to
school clubs, putting dinner on the table, getting stuck in traffic.
Monday through to Wednesdays are hard, and weekends on call
can be eventful, with the phone ringing any time of night or day:
a client needs milk, they got the time of day muddled, someone has been taken to hospital. Those weekends are a constant
intrusion into family life, and you get paid £152.

'I used to work in Sainsbury's, but I couldn't manage the night
shifts. I looked at care homes, but I couldn't do it. The routine
was so rushed and structured, you couldn't develop personal
relationships. In this job, the hours are long – sometimes twelve-
hour shifts, because there are gaps between visits when I am not
paid – but I love my clients and the hours suit me at the moment.
I usually earn about £850 a month.

'A couple I visit both have dementia. She is a German refu-
gee and she struggles to trust people. Her husband gets very
impatient for his food and she still wants to cook. I try not to
step on her toes, but it's tricky, because I only have an hour. It
requires real tact. Some clients are difficult, but someone has
to do it, and it's lucky it's me. It could be me in that situation

one day, and I would hope that someone would look after me well. I work so hard. I see it as a big loop. It's a way of putting something back in, replenishing the system. If I could do half of what my supervisor has done and have her memories, I will have done well. She is a real inspiration. She gives me advice about particular clients; she'll say things like, "If you talk about Ireland, she'll settle."

'People say, "Oh, you're just a carer," and at the school gate some parents look at me a bit funny when I say I am in domiciliary care. One parent thought I was a childminder, and I could see the shift in her face when I corrected her. I could never look after children. Elderly people have put so much into the world and you can learn from them. My sister, an ambulance driver, says she couldn't do my job, but I love it. I'm always thinking about my clients after I've left them.'

The company Sue works for emphasizes the quality of relationship, and charges above the market rate for it. Their marketing pamphlet mentions the word 'care' twenty-five times, and there are frequent references to compassion, respect, dignity and love: 'we regard it as a special privilege to look after people'. They recruit people who have 'hearts of gold' with 'a real caring nature, with empathy and a devotion to providing the highest quality care experience'.

On the website, I move from these descriptions to a tab with details of the business model, with graphs of the rising incidence of dementia and ageing demographics showing that it is recession-proof, with projections of likely turnover. As I browse, a chat window opens up, and 'Tim' offers to answer any questions. He suggests that one can grow a business with their model to have a million-pound turnover. 'What is the net profit on that?' I type back, but he says he can't answer that. With reason, I was to discover.

*

Nicola is just into her twenties, her face brimming with warmth and a ready smile. Dressed entirely in black, her nose and tongue are pierced, and her long hair is piled up on her head. She used to be a hairdresser, before joining the company two years ago, and it has been a revelation.

'At first, I was so scared I was shaking. I wondered how I would cope with the personal care, but now I'm fine with that. I wasn't a very confident person, but now I'm even a keyworker – introducing new carers – and an on-call supervisor. I couldn't have imagined I could ever do that, I've progressed so much. I always wanted to go into nursing, but I hated the brain work, I'm a hands-on type of person. But now I would like to go and work in a hospital one day.

'The pay is better than hairdressing, but the hours are very spread out. I work from 8 a.m. to 8.30 p.m., but am only paid for about six hours. In between my calls, I have another job doing administration for a shop. I probably do about twenty to thirty hours a week on the care job and make that up to a total of forty hours a week with both jobs. I'm on-call every other weekend, and I have to be in the office to rearrange visits, take and pass on messages. For the care job, I get £900–£1,000 after tax, unless my hours suddenly get cut – we are all on zero-hours contracts. If a client dies or goes into hospital, you can lose a lot of hours very suddenly. If there are extra calls, I'll usually do them. I once did seventeen days on the trot, but because I love my clients I didn't mind. I get better pay than most of my friends. You could earn a fortune if you worked all hours.

'I love the job and some of my clients are just great. The hour goes so quick. This morning, on one call, we were talking about football, and it wasn't like work. My clients feel like family. It's quite sad when you lose a client – they're like your nanny or granddad. People say, don't get too attached, but that's really hard. Most of the time I'm working on my own.

'One client has dementia and she gets upset, so I just give her a big hug and that cheers her up. She says to me, "You have such a warm heart." I think that's what these clients need. One client wouldn't let anyone else visit – only me. She died when I was on holiday – I felt very upset.

'There's sometimes a lot to fit into the hour, what with medication, assistance with washing, changing the bed, putting a wash on, washing up, making breakfast. After they have had a wash, they feel so much better. The personal care is important. Some of them just want a chat; you can't believe how happy that makes them. When you are starting out with a new client, you have to be alert and ready for whatever happens as you build up trust. I go home and I wonder if someone is OK – I worry about them.

'Some people think you're "just" a carer, but, trust me, we're the ones who have made the client's day. It's hard to explain that to people – but I'm not bothered. I know I'm making someone's life a lot better. I'm not being funny, but a lot of my friends are in hair and beauty, and do people really need their nails done or their hair coloured? There are a lot of elderly people, so I'm not going to be out of job. Soon, there'll only be care jobs.

'It can be draining, but it feels more satisfying to look after an elderly person. When people think it's all about personal care, I'd like them to see what we do – all the conversation and laughter. I've got one lady – I am seeing her three times tomorrow – and there won't be a moment of silence. Even when she is brushing her teeth, she chats. We have a giggle.'

A whiteboard in the company's offices had two lists of names. Staff who were leaving the company that month formed one list, while the other one, shorter, had the names of the clients who were leaving. The key task of the administrative team was to manage the relationship between the two. This was where 'warm hearts' were converted into numbers and hours. More than half the clients left every year, and the turnover of staff was just as high. The instability necessitated continuous marketing and recruitment, requiring full-time dedicated staff, a substantial cost for this small business. Recruitment was a struggle, with competition from better-paid jobs on supermarket checkouts with shorter hours and less responsibility. New clients were essential to ensure staff on zero-hours contracts had enough work, or they would leave. It was a delicate balancing act.

The nature of the work is unpredictable, and office staff worked long hours to manage the allocation of calls: one client had gone into hospital, one had sprained a wrist and needed more help; another client had a grandchild's birthday and would not be at home; another had a hospital appointment; a carer was sick, or their child was. There were 140 clients' lives to manage, 1,000 hours of care, and eighty-five carers on the books (mostly part time). There was no room for error; a missed call could be a matter of life and death. 'It burns people out,' admitted the managing director. It was Wednesday and there were 200 calls still to be allocated for the next fortnight. The following day, as I left for the evening, fifty calls over the weekend still needed staff.

John set up the company eight years ago. With a background in pharmacy, IT and insurance, he believed that he could set up a strong business to support his growing family. He wanted to develop an ethical business with high ideals around the quality of care. He mortgaged his house for the start-up capital. 'I've tried to do something with good intentions, and it's been painful, the most stressful thing I've ever done. I'm still working six days a week, with hugely long hours, perhaps sixty to seventy hours a week. There is a constant stream of staffing problems at every level of the organization; I'm on the fourth manager in seven years. We can't attract enough quality staff, and we can't keep them. It's bitty work compared to Tesco's. The carers take on big responsibilities for things like medicine, and for moving people and lifting with hoists. I'm told that there is a global shortage of care workers – as a society, we will have to turn to technology. We can't find carers prepared to go into the neighbouring rural areas: it is just not worth their while. Only one in ten of the younger people under forty stay for more than a year. It's always challenging to keep the business profitable, with constant juggling of staff and shifts. The office handles a steady stream of calls – Mrs X needs lunch, Mr Y needs new pills.

'The regulation and scrutiny have increased, and I have to recruit people just to manage the paperwork – every visit has to be recorded, with details of everything that has been done. We're just not trusted by the media or by government, and that's led to so much regulation. The new Care Certificate lists 250 standards, and each of them has to be signed off for each new carer with evidence.' Each recruit receives four days of training, which is not paid, but viewed as part of the interview process, a common practice across the sector. 'They are trying to professionalize the care work, and training now has to include mental-health conditions such as bipolar and schizophrenia, and basic life support, but the volume and intensity of training deters people; we had someone drop out recently who said if they were twenty years younger, they could deal with all the learning.

'I'm not sure professionalization is the right way to go to value this heart-based work. The Care Certificate will be a standard across hospital, care homes and domiciliary care, but the home-care companies say they are now training people who end up going into the NHS because the pay and conditions are better.'

The full-time recruiter, Jane, is on the lookout everywhere for people who have a reputation for being kind. In a moment of blunt honesty, she admits she couldn't do the job herself. 'What makes someone caring? It's the question I ask myself all the time,' she admits. 'Often someone has been stacking shelves at a supermarket and she's been told she's caring. But sometimes she will say she can do conversation, but not the personal care. That's a real problem for a lot of people. Continuity is really important – for the carer as well as the client. It is much easier to do personal care if you have a relationship with someone.

'We're looking for empathy, thoughtfulness and kindness. Where do all these qualities come from? Are they innate? It's really hard work recruiting, because the hours are long and unsociable. There is a lot of responsibility, and the clients' vulnerability and dependence are enormous. Often the carer is the only person to see the client on a regular basis.'

Sometimes Jane hits lucky. Tony worked in property maintenance for most of his life, and an advert in a post office after he had retired piqued his interest. After several years working as a carer, he still can't believe how much he loves the work.

'I wish I'd done care work all my life. I've never had the satisfaction from work that I get from seeing one of my clients. I love the people. You doubt yourself in the early part of the job, and I would take things home with me and not sleep half the night, but I'm more experienced now, and there is some good support in the office. I've had people with dementia who can be violent or rude, but I think, There but for the grace of God go I. I don't judge the person. I just get this little sense of satisfaction that I've done everything I can for that person if I can leave them with a smile on their face. My wife says she has never seen me so happy. My daughter says that I have changed so much, and that I'm more relaxed and funny.

'I see one client six days a week. I looked after her husband, and before he died he asked me to look after her, and that's what I will do. I do some light housework for her, and massage her legs and put on her stockings. I'm not bothered by this being considered women's work – it's not just women who need to clean up. I found the personal care very straightforward – it's part and parcel of the job and I just deal with it.

'I work nearly every day. I get up at 6 a.m. and leave at 7.45 for the first call. It does take a certain kind of person to do this job. I get the impression that some people think it will be easy, and that it is just sitting with someone for a cup of tea, but that's a big mistake. The most important thing is to make that person feel at ease with you, comfortable and look forward to you going back.

'I don't do pity – you can't do that. When I was ill, I didn't want pity. I've had serious illnesses, and they gave me an understanding of suffering. I almost died and was very fortunate to survive. Life is very precious, and since then I have had a very different outlook on life. I do the job because I love it, not because of the money – it is pretty poor compared to the skills you need. I've bumped into old acquaintances, and they can't believe I'm a carer. If I had done it years ago, it would have made me a better person. My wife would say I'm not the man she married. I was an awkward character, a jealous swine. The clients have changed me so much – they've humbled me. Most of them have major problems, and yet very few of them mention them; they have such courage and forbearance.

'It's a whole world I have stepped into and it's been so rich. That one advert changed my life and continues to do so. I have no intention of stopping, and I'll continue as long as I can. The one downside of the job is when people die – more so than I can even tell you. I still take the job home with me. At the moment things are stable, but in the past I've been awake many times worrying, wondering what I can do. I just can't switch off. It's like these clients – I call them friends – are part of my extended family.'

Pamela, a former mental-health nurse, left the NHS frustrated by the burden of paperwork, but was drawn back to care work and took the job because she liked the autonomy.

'I do struggle with the lack of communication in this kind of home care. As nurses, we had loads of meetings and risk assessments all the time. I used to work with very inspiring people. It's more tricky in this job: you are on your own, and when you visit a client, you only have an entry in the journal to go on. It's very task-oriented and I found it quite frustrating to start with. On visits, I use a lot of my skills as a mental-health nurse, and I do wonder how others are coping. One particular lady was very distressed and was trying to leave the building. Bringing in more reflective practices would help with staff retention, I think.

'There was a client recently who was dying, and we had to double up (two staff were needed). It was wonderful to work with a really good carer, and I really enjoyed it. They were respectful and loving to the family. The client died at home, very settled, calm and comfortable. It made me feel really good.

'I do think it's a valuable thing to do. I've done enough work on dementia to know the impact of good care in slowing down the disease. I've always had the feeling that I have to give back. I've had a lovely life. That's how my dad felt. I know what I'm doing now is important – there is an inner motivation which comes from that knowledge and confidence in what you do. It's innate, instinctive. I grew up in a very loving family. My father did a lot of voluntary work, and I've always done voluntary work with the elderly.

'I don't get too emotionally involved. I know it's part of the client's journey in life. There is always something to do to improve things and to help. I never underestimate the impact I can make; every single member of staff, qualified or unqualified, can make a difference.'

The biggest drawback of the work, she says, is the pay. She admits it can make her cross. 'It works out at only £8.50 an hour. My daughter had a part-time job at Sainsbury's before university, and she did eight hours straight and earnt a lot more.

*

John's final comment was gloomy. 'This is much harder than any other industry I have worked in; people in the insurance industry get paid twice as much for half the responsibility.' He is troubled and admits, 'We're taking advantage of people's sense of vocation to care.'

Stressful and precarious, the business puts immense pressure on the office staff who have to handle multiple forms of anxiety – of clients, their families and the staff. Apart from the annual Christmas party, the carers rarely meet each other. There is little, if any, sense of a shared collective purpose, and no institutional or organizational structure to inspire or provide solidarity to underpin individual effort. Even the language is problematic: the supervisor confessed she didn't like the way care was referred to as an 'industry'. It was a vocation, she insisted, and the work reflected her strongly held values on the worth of each human being.

The struggles described by John, Sue and Nicola – for a viable small business, for decent working hours and pay – reflect a crisis that has deepened dramatically in recent years. Thousands of similar small companies are engaged in this kind of precarious hard work as the market for domiciliary care teeters close to collapse. Those with local-authority contracts have been under even more pressure, because budgets cannot stretch to the minimum sustainable price for home care. As a result, companies are walking away from the contracts; according to one survey, more than half of social-care providers have handed back contracts to the local-authority areas and many more fear they will have to do so in the future. The brunt of cuts in social-care budgets has fallen in home care and other community services which support the elderly at home, such as day centres (30 per cent cuts since 2009, compared to just 4 per cent in residential care). Two of the largest national providers of domiciliary care announced they would no longer take any publicly funded clients. People are paying for their own care at a cost currently estimated at around £1 billion a year. Those who can't afford to pay end up with visits of thirty minutes from overstretched private companies scraping by on inadequate local-authority funding, or they are amongst the 1.4 million estimated to have been excluded from the care system altogether through tightened criteria. They have to manage for themselves, leaning on friends and family for help. Complaints about home care to the ombudsman have risen by a third in three years, and the fallout from this threadbare system lands on the NHS: delays in discharge have increased sharply since 2010 (so-called bed blocking); the single biggest cause is that patients are having to wait for a home-care package to be put in place.

In another company, home-care visits were fifteen minutes. Kelly was shocked. 'I was very green and willing; they trusted me with very vulnerable people after only three hours of basic health-and-safety training. I had no training in moving and lifting, and it's left me with historic back pain. I wasn't paid for travel time. It was an eye-opener: the vulnerability of these elderly people having to rely on a stranger. The clients didn't know me, and I was coming into their house to wake them up. I might be assisting them at their most vulnerable, helping them get to the toilet, without ever having been introduced or having met them before. Sometimes there wasn't even time to make them a hot drink in the morning – as a carer, you always want to offer that. Luxury was a thirty-minute visit. There was no time for eye contact, and certainly no time to get to know the person and their story. You often had to give medication, and write up notes. It was scary – a very negative experience. My shift was 7 a.m. to 3 p.m., but I would work sometimes until 8 p.m. because I was always behind. Later I discovered that my insurance stopped at 3 p.m., and after that it was at my own risk.

'I worried about people – had they had a hot meal? Did the doctor come? I took all the worries home with me. I went down to six-and-half stone, and I wasn't sleeping. It lasted eighteen months, but it felt like a marathon. I wanted to explain to the manager why I was leaving, and that this wasn't the way to do care. I'm true to my star sign, Libris – Justice – and when I feel passionate, I have to speak up. The manager told me that it was all about cost – that was what social services could afford.

'I was a whistle-blower. Sometimes we had to double up, and I was shocked at the way carers spoke to a patient, as if they were a child – things like, "Come on, don't be silly, Betty, I haven't got time" – or spoke about them as if they weren't there. It was belittling, and stripped them of dignity.'

Another home-care worker, Blessing, still finds the memory of her work with another home-care company difficult, and at one point in our interview she broke down in tears.

'A lot of people literally pleaded with me to stay for a moment, just to have a cup of tea. I would try to stay for as long as I could, perhaps five minutes more. I always felt bad walking out, knowing that the client might not see anyone until the next carer. It felt very mechanical: you go in and you do your job and then you had to leave. I saw eight to twelve people a day; a lot of them had dementia.

'I knew nothing about dementia when I started, and was startled at first. I went in to one gentleman to organize his breakfast and personal care, then a few hours later I was back, and he didn't remember me from one visit to the next, and would get irritable. My training had been very basic. He never got to the point of knowing me, but on one of my visits, as a way of calming him down, I asked if I could sit down and have a cup of tea and a sandwich with him. He loved that, and we sat and talked, and I asked him about his life. Then he said something really amazing: "No matter how hard things get, you must face them with a smile." He was looking past me at the garden. I loved the way he said it. It didn't just roll off his tongue, it was thoughtful.

'The care agency was all about money; they would tell me who to visit and that was it. I worked on my own most of the time. Once, I noticed an old lady in her nineties had bruises on her arms. She told me that her previous carers had been rough. She was very co-operative – I couldn't see how the bruises could have happened. I was distraught. She asked if I could come back again, and I said I would try my hardest. I called the office and told them about the bruises, and they said they would deal with it. I was crying, so I called my mother. I was in so much emotional pain.'

Blessing took a deep breath as she apologized and wiped tears away. The agency didn't allocate her to the lady again, and she never heard anything more. 'It was such a sad day. On the phone, my mother told me: that's why people need someone like you. She told me that it is the type of work you do with mercy in your heart for these people.'

Between her tears, she added, 'It was the vulnerability of the lady and the way she asked me to come back. My mother is one of the most caring people I have ever met. She is very religious, she's a Roman Catholic. I'm not religious, but I've tried to adopt the way she copes with things. Forgiveness is a big part of her life.'

After our interview, I looked up the care agency Blessing had worked for; it was a franchise, but the web links repeatedly broke. They had been subject to an investigation by the Care Quality Commission and seemed to have disappeared.

When I asked Blessing why she has worked in care, she laughed: 'I just love people, and I always try to put myself in their shoes.'

She had just started a new job as an activities coordinator in a residential home, and, to her delight, it gave her time to talk to the residents. 'I've made a point of going round to find out all their interests, and already, in the five weeks I've been there, I've made changes. One resident hadn't left his bedroom for over a year. The carers told me that he was sometimes aggressive. I introduced myself and he was a bit irritable, but I just smiled and asked about his hobbies. He said he liked opera and musicals, so I started singing a song from *Cats*. He told me I was punching above my station.' Blessing threw her head back, laughing again. 'So I replied that he'd better teach me. I showed him how I could find opera on my phone. He gave me a list of songs. We found *"Je crois entendre encore"* by Bizet. He was sitting in his wheelchair with tears of joy running down his cheek and waving his hand in the air to the music.

'All the other carers were amazed. He's a lot more patient and kind with the other staff now. He talked to me about his background and growing up. Every single day I make a differ-ence – that's job satisfaction. I feel I am doing my job well. I make a difference for people who have no family and I do it with love – that's the word I use – I tell each one of them that I love them. I want them to feel happy, even if it's only for one hour. Today we were playing music, and an elderly guy started crying uncontrollably. He said that his family and friends had all abandoned him and that he had no one. I told him, "We're your family now, we're here for you."

'This work makes me happy. A lot of my friends ask how I do this work, cleaning old people's bums. I just picture I am doing it for my mum or someone else I love. Everyone needs to be cared for; these things don't faze me. When I was growing up, people looked out for the elderly, and young people respected them, but it's not like that now. A lot of elderly people have been forgotten about. We've lost a sense of connection with other people. When people's interactions are on a more technological basis, you lose basic human compassion.

'People think that what I do is menial labour. I don't care two
monkeys. I know what I do and that's what counts. It serves
people in a way other people might not be able to understand.
I'm guided by the goodness instilled by my mother.'

Kelly also moved on to residential care. 'The care home looked
nice, with flower arrangements, and I was seduced by the
environment, but it was very regimented, like a conveyor belt:
waking people up, helping them with personal care. It was
always about the quickest, easiest thing to do. I noticed how
carers would talk to each other while they were feeding someone, and there was no eye contact with the client. At night, the
bells went all the time and one caregiver unplugged the bell
on a patient – I whistle-blew on that, but I don't think they did
anything. The worst thing was seeing a carer washing the face
of a client who was still asleep.

'I worked in two or three homes. At tea breaks I was always
alone, because I kept complaining about things. I got scared
that the other caregivers might set me up in a situation in which
I could be found at fault and accused of abuse. I knew they
wanted to get rid of me.

'I had two successes in those years which I will always laugh
about. The cook walked out one Christmas and I ended up
cooking for forty-eight people on Boxing Day. I also managed
to do a charity bake-off, with a couple of residents helping in
the kitchen. We opened up the gardens, which were beautiful
but rarely used. The residents loved it all – they lit up and I saw
a different way of doing things.

'I asked myself, why do I see people walk into a care home and
then end up doing nothing but sitting around or being wheeled
about? It was because it was easier for the care workers. I knew
I liked this kind of work; I made a difference to someone. It's a
very personal thing to make someone feel verified as a human

being. Your well-being is only as good as the care you receive. I was always drawn to older people. I find them fascinating and they have so much to tell you about. One of our clients created the postcode system, another worked at Bletchley. They have had amazing lives – why wouldn't you want to listen? I've been taught so many things by my clients. Looking back, I think it started with my grandparents. I spent a lot of my childhood with them. My grandfather did lots of charity work – meals on wheels, that kind of thing. My paternal grandmother was a very caring person, and nothing was ever too much trouble for her.'

'After my experience in the care homes, I felt my heart had been shattered. One person can't make a difference, I was fighting a tide. Unless someone at the top makes changes, I couldn't do anything. I told myself to turn my heart off and I took a job in a shop. It was a year before I got over the guilt of not doing the care job. All of this care work – I see it as a profession – is an investment for myself for when I am old.

The care-home sector (nursing and residential) is gripped by a different kind of crisis to that in home care. The sector is growing significantly, with an estimated annual revenue of nearly £16.9 billion. New homes are being built and there is a lot of money to be made; overseas investors see rich and reliable pickings, not least from the steady flow of government funding, and 80 per cent of all care-home property deals, 2016–18, involved overseas investors. But the sector is dominated by a few large operators owned by private-equity companies, who have loaded them up with massive debt and constructed elaborate group structures which often conceal their true costs. These deeply unstable financial enterprises have long caused concern. In 2011 the then-biggest operator, Southern Cross, failed, threatening the stability of 750 homes with 17,000 residents. The case was widely covered in the media and there was

deep alarm, but it was not sufficient to prevent a highly lever-
aged deal in 2012, when a private-equity group bought another
major operator, Four Seasons. It tottered from crisis to crisis,
with injections of cash for crippling interest payments, until it
finally went into administration in April 2019, as had long been
predicted. The biggest care-home company, HC-One, with 349
homes, has an estimated £500 million in borrowing; it is part
of a Cayman Islands-based group of forty-three companies,
of which six are offshore. The *Financial Times* calculated in
2019 that accounts for the four biggest care-home companies,
running 900 homes between them, with 55,000 residents, had
accumulated levels of debt which required £40,000 per bed
annually in interest charges alone. Such companies complain
that meagre local-authority funding is the cause of the crisis
in the sector – and there is an element of truth in this – but
an even more significant cause is the financialization of the
privatized care sector, whereby property assets are separated
from running costs, and then used as collateral for borrowing
money. Care homes have become financial instruments to generate profit. The result is deeply unstable: in 2017 commercial
analysts estimated that a third of the UK's bed capacity in residential care was at risk of closing in the next five years. That
may not be of great concern to the surviving operators – they
could then push prices up.

The market is grotesquely distorting an essential service.
The number of residential beds has been in steady decline
since 2010, but, even more seriously, there is significant regional
variation; Hull, for example, lost a third of its beds in the five
years up to 2019, and York lost a third in three years. Across the
country 'care deserts' are appearing. In affluent areas, shortages
of staff restrict provision, while homes are forced to close in
poorer parts of the country because most residents' fees are paid
by local authorities, at a rate which does not cover full costs.

Meanwhile, the demand from an ageing population continues to grow, outstripping supply, particularly of nursing-home places.

Older people are caught in the epicentre of the crisis caused by a deficit of funding, organizational culture, relationship, time and attention. A succession of governments have tolerated financial gambling with the essential service of residential care, which depends on the understanding of care of workers like Sue, Blessing, Tony and Kelly. Empathy and sleepless nights from people like them are subsidising a casino in which the chips are the well-being of thousands of vulnerable older people.

This dysfunction is widely acknowledged across all political parties. It erupts intermittently, grabbing headlines, provoking alarm and politicians' anguished pledges that something will be done. NHS leaders have repeatedly urged action on social care, because the knock-on effects on health services are so significant; without effective social care, older people turn up in A & E departments, and return more frequently to hospital and stay longer, putting pressure on NHS budgets. Since the Royal Commission into long-term care in 1999, there have been a succession of major reports (Wanless in 2006, Dilnott in 2011, Barker in 2014), but they have not been translated into the ambitious overhaul of funding and provision that has been repeatedly and urgently recommended. Instead, there have been a few piecemeal initiatives designed to ease the pressure on the NHS; otherwise, the issue has become a political football. Theresa May's attempt to grasp the nettle in the 2017 election was widely blamed for contributing to her poor result at the ballot box. In the 2019 election both Labour and Conservatives pledged action: Labour made a bold and expensive commitment to extending free personal care for over sixty-fives, at a cost of £6 billion; the Conservative manifesto promises were vague. In a joint report two of the country's biggest health think tanks bitterly lamented that 'England remains one of the few major advanced countries that has not reformed the way it funds long-term care in response to an ageing population.' They warned that the gap between need and resources has ballooned, reaching £2.9 billion in 2019, and that public spending on adult social care has fallen to less than 1 per cent of GDP, behind many other European countries. Scandinavian countries spend more than twice as much; Germany, Italy and Lithuania are substantially more generous.

One of the more thoughtful inquiries into care work, the Cavendish Review in 2013, considered how best to ensure the 1.3 million workers in hospitals and social care look after their clients with compassion. 'Helping an elderly person to eat and swallow, bathing someone with dignity and without hurting them, communicating with someone with early onset dementia; doing these things with intelligent kindness, dignity, care and respect requires skill. Doing so alone in the home of a stranger, when the district nurse has left no notes, and you are only being paid to be there for thirty minutes, requires considerable maturity and resilience.' It warned that care workers were taking on increasingly challenging tasks, 'yet their training is hugely variable. Some employers are not meeting their basic duty to ensure their staff are competent. Some staff were given a DVD to watch at home before being sent straight out to the front line.'

In the conclusion, it stated, 'An inescapable fact is that good caring takes time. It will not be possible to build a sustainable, caring, integrated health and social-care system on the backs of domiciliary care workers who have to travel long distances on zero-hours contracts, to reach people who have to see multiple different faces each week. Local authorities must start to commission for outcomes, not by the minute – which is a false economy when so many staff are quitting.' The chair of the review, Camilla Cavendish, admitted, 'I could never do the jobs these women do, let alone do it with the glow they bring to their work. I have come away from this project thinking that our society is incredibly lucky to have so many people with a dedication to caring. But I also fear that if we continue to take them for granted, if we do not fix dysfunctional systems of commissioning and regulation, we may find as we grow old that they are not there to look after us.' One of the Cavendish recommendations, a new system of Care Certificates, was introduced in 2015 – adding to John's woes with more bureaucracy – but the more radical recommendation to change the commissioning model away from time to tasks has made no headway.

The political stalemate on the subject (exacerbated by the preoccupation with Brexit since 2016) entails deliberately ignoring how other government policies increase the strain on social care. The introduction of the National Living Wage (phased in from 2016 to 2020), while bringing a much-needed improvement in wage levels for thousands of care workers, is adding even more pressure on companies like John's. By 2020 it will inflate local-authority annual costs by £800 million, when demand is rising due to the ageing population, and there is no increase in central-government funding. Local authorities face further costs from equal-pay claims for historic underpayment of care work; for example, Glasgow council is due to pay £500 million to home-care workers affected by discriminatory pay policies. The council's head of social work was reported as saying that up to 40 per cent could use their settlement payout to take early retirement, crippling the city's home-care capacity. Equal-pay claims pending in other local authorities, with a similar age profile of care workers, could have a comparable impact.

Another characteristic of this bizarre policy landscape is the ungrounded ambition; the 2014 Care Act created new, admirable responsibilities for local authorities, but with no further funding. It has ratcheted up expectations even further, without consideration of how they would be paid for; only a pitiful 2 per cent of directors of social services said they could fulfil the act's new requirements. This is zombie policy, empty of meaning, provoking untold frustration for those expected to implement it, as well as those hoping to benefit.

Care for older people has suffered from a toxic combination of chronic underinvestment and politicians' reluctance to spell it out to the electorate: new money is needed, and that must come either from increased taxes or from personal contributions. Increasingly, many have been paying for private care, but much of the public still believes in William Beveridge's boast of care from 'cradle to grave', and expects care to be free at the point of need. All too often, the reality is a shock to relatives and patients, and what continually baffles is the unclear boundary between healthcare (which is still free and available) and social care (which is often not free and sometimes not even available). A patient suffering from cancer can receive free healthcare, but a patient with dementia may receive nothing. The distinction can be deeply distressing.

What is still only dimly understood is that under successive Thatcher governments in the 1980s, the NHS was safeguarded (to some extent), but social care was not, and was privatized by stealth; local-authority provision shrank dramatically and the private sector expanded. Social care was rigorously means-tested (currently, you are expected to pay if you have assets over £23,250), and the proportion paying for their care has steadily climbed ever since.

The public must bear some share of the blame for the mess; many are as reluctant as the politicians to face the issue squarely. The lack of interest is striking, given that everyone ages, and social care is a service on which many may come to depend. Research in the US – where insurance companies have a keen interest – estimates that 70 per cent of those turning sixty-five will need some form of long-term care, with a sharp difference between men (58 per cent) and women (79 per cent), as women care for their male partners and then live longer. On average, women will need 3.7 years of care and men will need 2.2 years, but the averages obscure the wide variation: one third will not need long-term care at all, while 20 per cent will need it for more than five years. With figures like these, old age is a lottery in which some win through, and others will need care costing hundreds of thousands of pounds; many voters appear to be gambling on being in the former category.

The refusal to recognize the issue is rooted in a deeply entrenched aversion to the inevitability of ageing, and the relationships of dependence it brings. This fear seems not just to contaminate the entire policy debate, but to seep into the valuing of the work of caring for older people. When I was on the oncology ward shadowing nurses, there was a brief, poignant exchange between a nursing auxiliary and a woman who had come in for a procedure to treat ovarian cancer. She looked very scared, and as the auxiliary was making her comfortable, he asked her what her job was. A healthcare assistant in a care home, she replied, adding that 'It's not a proper job like yours.' Taken aback, he insisted that their work was comparable, but she disagreed. She just wiped bums, she said.

At the top end of the home-care market, agencies can provide a carer to live in the client's home. It is extremely expensive. But even in this luxury model, the work is isolated, very demanding and deeply demoralizing. Claire found herself with no money after studying for a master's and ended up working for six years for a big agency which recruits from abroad (mainly white South Africans).

'I loathed the work. Friends and people I meet don't ask me about it; I think it's partly to save me from discomfort and embarrassment, because it's low-status work – as if it's shameful.

When I was working, someone once addressed me as "Carer" – I no longer had a name. It is not even very well paid, and there's no sick or holiday pay, travel time isn't paid; it worked out at about £72–£100 a day before tax, but after time off to rest, it didn't work out at much. My bookings were all over the country. Ten hours a day, with a break of two hours in the afternoon if you were lucky.

'Clients felt entitled to comment on everything – the way I dressed, what I ate. I lost count of the number of arguments I had over what I could eat for breakfast if I didn't want to eat the same as the client. I'm an adult with my own preferences. To others, it was simply a commercial transaction in which I was not recognized as a person. I felt my identity was erased.

'My first client was known as the "wicked witch of the south". She was hugely wealthy and there were photos of her as a debutante, but the previous carer warned me she would not feed me. I was so frightened that I took food with me. She was downright mean. I worked really hard, and felt I had cracked it: I kept everything spotless, but she found a small mark on the bin. She told me I was disgusting. She had grown up with servants. I managed to stick it out, and the daughter even asked me to come back, but it was humiliating. The sense of rage I felt was sometimes unbelievable. Often, I wanted to just walk out.

'I would work for a client for two weeks and then take a week off, but I couldn't always afford to take the week off, so I sometimes had to work for longer. You could be interrupted through the night, especially when the client had severe dementia. One lady would get very distressed, but she couldn't communicate, so you didn't know what the matter was. The previous carer just said, "Be firm with her," but I could see that was crazy. If large portions of the map have been rubbed away, you have to build a relationship with a person very quickly. The carer had explained how to take her to the bathroom, but the client started screaming. She kept calling her husband's name. She pushed me out of the way. She was tiny but very strong, and she managed to get to the top of the stairs. I was terrified one of the family might find us there. She was only half-dressed. I tried to find a way to calm her down and we stayed there for over forty-five minutes. I gradually moved her to a chair and got her trousers on.

'I managed two weeks with that client, but it was very hard. I left a very detailed note for the next carer to give them an idea. I can understand why some carers snap and are rough when they get to the point where they can't cope. It's intense and lonely work. I have a qualification in psychotherapy, so I have skills, but it's unbelievably exhausting and hugely demanding.

'Sometimes it was satisfying when I worked out the needs of a client, but there is no one to share that success with, and no external validation. It was the hardest thing I've ever done. Once, I went in to wake a person with dementia and she hit me in the face. She was frightened, but you need a developed mental model to keep empathy, because it cuts to the core of who you are. It can be frightening. Another time, the previous carer told me at handover that the client had attacked someone with scissors, so I mustn't ever turn my back on her. I rang the daughter. There was a long pause and then she told me that her mother was capricious and often attacked her carers. She told me that if I was attacked, I should go into the garden and call the police. I had told the agency that I couldn't deal with violence, but I was worried that if I complained about a job, I wouldn't get bookings or I'd get difficult ones. The agency was very commercially oriented, and always took the client's side. There was no meaningful support. In the agency office, no one had actually done the job and they didn't know anything about it.

'One client with dementia had a urinary tract infection. She was waking me fifteen or twenty times in the night and I had to help her with the toilet. It was physically demanding to pull her up the bed. As soon as I got back to bed, she rang again. That went on for four nights, and I wasn't coping. A gardener noticed this and was so worried about me that he rang the agency, and they sent another person to cover the nights.

'At first, I wasn't assertive enough. Clients felt they could lose their temper with me. I came from a therapeutic background, and I was not used to laying down boundaries, such as, "You don't speak to me like that." Sometimes clients are just winding you up and being capricious. There is a lot of daytime TV and a lot of repetitive question patterns. They were often dyed-in-the-wool Tories, people whose life experience was different from mine in every conceivable way.

'I did have a few clients that I loved. Polly and I had a similar sense of humour and enjoyed the absurd. She was very clever. It was like putting a six-year-old to bed, it was so lovely to be with her. I got to know her whole family. With dementia, people don't lose who they are; sometimes it refines the core of the person, and can be exquisitely beautiful: Polly was so much herself. We had an incredibly strong intuitive bond. It was like the relationship between a mother and child, or with a partner. Polly muddled her words, but I could still understand, and we always got each other's jokes.

'In the end, I left. I just couldn't take it anymore. Sometimes clients abuse carers. I could see why a carer snaps: "There but for the grace of God, go I." It's badly paid, with long hours, is poorly understood and has no professional standing. When you say, "I'm a carer," the conversation dries up. I found it very shaming – embarrassing – to be educated and middle class and to have descended to the level of carer. I'm still recovering a sense of self six months on. I am trying to come back into the world.'

After the interview, Claire emailed: 'Thank you so much for listening to me. Having someone reflect back the layered and multiple nature of the erasure of personhood I experienced was enormously helpful and kind. Like feminism, having a word for the problem can be empowering.'

There is no tradition of ageing wisely in the West, unlike in many Asian and African cultures where age has prestige, status and is associated with wisdom, suggests Chris Phillipson, a sociologist of ageing. Age has been ridiculed as 'dotage'; Shakespeare described it as a second childhood. The tragedy of *King Lear* is triggered by the ageing king's narcissism and stupidity. Charles Dickens often depicted elderly characters as petty dictators, controlling the family wealth and imposing cruel marriage choices. Phillipson quotes an extraordinary outburst from the great social scientist Richard Titmuss in 1942 as symptomatic of a deep anxiety in British culture; fearing that an ageing society would bring social progress to a grinding halt, Titmuss declared: 'we are up against something fundamental, something vast and almost terrifying in its grim relentless development'. Society would 'lose the mental attitude that is essential for social progress, the greater intelligence, courage, power of initiative, and qualities of creative imagination not usually found in the aged'. In 1949 the Royal Commission on Population lamented that 'it is the fact that (with some exceptions) the old consume without producing which differentiates them from the active population and makes them a factor reducing the average standard of living of the community'. In short, they were a burden, a drain on the country's resources. Such attitudes give some indication of what might lie behind a terrible history of care for older people in the UK.

The reality is that the UK has never had a system of long-term care for the elderly; the current predicament is the continuation of a long trend of neglect, indifference and lack of funding. The crisis is now reaching unprecedented proportions as this

is confronted by an ageing demographic and rising expectations from a wealthy consumer society. In the early twentieth
century welfare was preoccupied with social problems such as
unemployment and sickness among working-age men, and with
pensions for the elderly. Those needing long-term care were
fewer in number and, if too poor to pay for their care, were left
to languish in the punitive regimes of workhouses. During the
Second World War, hospital beds were needed for war casualties,
and older people were unceremoniously moved into environments described by Charles Webster, the official historian of
the NHS, as little better than concentration camps. Post-war,
Beveridge's rhetoric of care was never matched by the necessary
'enthusiasm, precision or a sense of priority', as one historian put
it. With little faith that much could be done for older people with
chronic conditions and mental illness, residential care was cus-
todial rather than therapeutic. Conditions in asylums horrified
a succession of politicians, including Enoch Powell and Richard
Crossman, yet, as Webster concludes, 'the elderly bore their
disappointment with dignity and general public indignation was
slow to materialize'. By the end of the 1950s, out of 6.7 million
older people, 300,000 lived in institutions and 60,000 were in
what were known as 'back wards'. These were often part of a
general hospital; they were underfunded, overcrowded and there
was little medical supervision (one consultant admitted he had
1,500 patients under his sole charge). Beds were lined up only
inches apart in wards that housed up to sixty people. Many of
these old hospital buildings dated from Victorian times, with
little heating – one researcher noted that urine froze in the
bedpans – and erratic electricity. Peter Townsend, a researcher
at the London School of Economics, captured the desolation:
'It is not just the appearance, the coarseness to the touch, the
noise or the impenetrable silence, but the smell of neglect that
remains imprinted on the mind: the sweet but slightly rotting

smell of an assortment of bewildered human beings who exist in claustrophobic proximity like wrinkling apples spaced fractionally apart in a dark cupboard.' The Labour politician Richard Crossman visited one of the most infamous institutions, Friern Barnet, in the mid-1960s, and was left 'subdued and shaken by the stench and the soaking walls, [and] the treatment of helpless, incontinent and usually relationless patients'.

Another visitor to Friern Barnet in 1964 was Barbara Robb, a flamboyant, well-connected Hampstead psychotherapist; she was so horrified that she dedicated the next ten years to a vociferous and high-profile campaign with lasting impacts. In 1967 Robb published her book, *Sans Everything*, an edited collection of contributions from nurses and social workers and a diary Robb had written of her visits to Friern Barnet. She described how patients had uniform haircuts, institutional clothing, and were deprived of all personal possessions in a routine known as 'stripping': spectacles, hearing aids and dentures were taken away to ensure they were not lost or broken. Deliberate cruelty was rare, but rough handling could come close; teasing, slapping and swearing were commonplace. Patients had no privacy and were bathed in groups on a 'production line', and toileting could be in full view of the ward.

Robb's book was a bestseller and caused a public outcry, but the government response was dismissive. Crossman admitted in his diaries that she was a 'terrible danger' to the government, and likened her to a 'bomb' which 'had to be defused'. Robb's work was picked up by ITV's *World in Action* and the resulting film of Powick Hospital's back ward, F13, presented a horrifying picture. She was finally vindicated by the findings of an inquiry into Cardiff's Ely Hospital, where a young barrister (Geoffrey Howe, later to be a key figure in the Thatcher governments) made his name by upholding allegations of neglect and poor management. By the time Robb died of cancer in 1974, her campaigning had contributed to the creation of a new special-ism – psychiatric geriatrics – an inspectorate and an ombudsman system for complaints. Eventually it contributed to the closure of the back wards and huge asylums, and the development of smaller units and a shift of policy towards community care.

Likened to other upper-class women reformers such as Elizabeth Fry and Florence Nightingale, Robb has had a fraction of their fame. 'For one woman to suddenly do so much in such a short period – and tragically to die so soon – is a remarkable story,' commented the social researcher Brian Abel Smith. She was one of the pioneers of a new style of campaigning on social issues, adroitly using the media, and setting up a pressure group to lobby government, which has since been powerful in the history of care. The pattern of scandal, outcry and govern-ment response has been evident in a succession of cases, most importantly at the Mid Staffordshire NHS Foundation Trust in the 2000s. Other instances include Winterbourne View, a care home for people with learning disabilities, where in 2012 footage showed shocking ill treatment. Inspections, widespread use of CCTV and more regulation have been introduced to improve standards, but the prime drivers of abuse – excessive workloads, poor training, low staffing – persist. As one study acknowledged, 'psychological experiments have shown time and time again that we are all capable of neglect at least if not active abuse', as a person's behaviour is affected by environment and culture in what is known as 'situational attribution'.

Increased regulation has added to the burden of paperwork. The same study identified 100 separate items of paperwork that must be completed regularly in care homes, and the study's author, John Kennedy, said that 'the most startling finding' was that the quality of the care home's paperwork had come to be rated more highly than the quality of care; staff were assessed and promoted for their ability to complete forms. Managers told him that paperwork took up a fifth of their time. After thirty years of working in care for the elderly, Kennedy lamented that the sector has stumbled from crisis to crisis, stricken by an inexcusable indifference and plagued by low pay and poor working conditions: 'Why, if care for our most vulnerable and frail is so important, so fundamental to our sense of righteousness, do we treat those who provide care so badly?'

The residents in the care home are mostly women, and sit in a circle of armchairs in the day room. One has a beautifully alert face and, dressed in her bright pink cardigan, she glows with delight. 'Thank you so much for coming.' Manners often seem to be the last thing to be lost. 'Nice to meet you.' She smiles at me as if she were a duchess.

'Your hand is so cold,' she exclaims, as she keeps hold. 'Warm it on a man's bottom.' She roars with laughter at her ribald comment. She has one prominent front tooth when she smiles.

Over the course of several months, I volunteered for several projects working with older people; I wanted to understand better the task of caring for an older person with dementia, and I trained in hand massage; as the disease erodes comprehension, touch can be a more effective way to communicate reassurance.

Sharon mumbles something which I can't grasp, but her face breaks into a toothless smile. Her eyelids are hovering – she seems to be falling asleep – but when I ask her if she is enjoying the massage, they flick open. 'Ooh, its lovely,' she says.

I move on to an Asian lady, sitting very upright. Every now and then, she flings out a defiant cry across the room. She has a scarf tied around her head. I have no way of knowing what she thinks of anything. One minute she is dismissive and I think I am irritating her, the next she seems to soften. In contrast, Barbara smiles cheerfully. She has a box of jelly babies beside her and admits shyly that she likes them. Despite the smile and the eye contact, she is very confused. I ask about a hand massage and she looks at her hands, holds them out. She has very long thin fingers and she gnaws on one.

'I could eat half my finger,' she says. Throughout the time we spend together, she repeats anxiously, 'I won't get into trouble,' and, 'That won't get me into trouble.' All that is left of her memory is some history of authority and trouble.

Another woman is sobbing from the other side of the room. After asking the care assistant, I go over to offer a massage. She is talking in an inaudible voice and I lean over to try to make sense. She seems very distressed. Suddenly, sharp as a bell, she asks, 'What are you doing standing over me?' I beat a hasty retreat. Mary seems the most coherent. She was asleep, her hair awry, when I arrived, but after a while she puts on her headscarf, and talks to me about how she is going out. 'Is that all right? Will there be any left?' It's not clear what she is referring to. She's very sorry but she doesn't have time, she says, but thank you for coming. Maybe next time.

The extreme old seem to have so much time. It is poured into their lap, day after day. They are the ones rich in the stuff, while everyone caring for them is acutely short of it. It creates an impossible and frustrating imbalance. Everyone longs for more time except those who sit and wait for their next meal. Yet this abundance is poised on the edge – at any moment, time might run out.

The home appeared to be well run and there were plenty of staff. But the quiet routine seemed to amplify the sense of surplus, of unneeded human beings and of unwanted time. I saw visitors only once during the weeks I was there. The elderly residents were like a group of people cast adrift after a shipwreck; they seemed bewildered to have arrived at this moment in their lives, struggling to make sense of the strangers who moved around them. How do you make relationships in this world of aged women with their exaggerated bodies – either near skeletal, fragile as a cobweb, or their ample contours spilling over their armchair.

The following week, Shirley was wandering around the room, very agitated. She repeatedly came up to me, then she wandered over to Mary and took her cake, tried to take her drink.

Christine was much more confused this time. 'Where is Mummy and Daddy?' she kept asking. 'I haven't seen my mummy for ages.' She looked utterly lost. I stroked her hand and she seemed to like it, but then she wanted to show me a folded napkin. She handed it over as if it were infinitely precious.

Mary was on good form. I sat down beside her and we chatted about her bright pink flounced skirt and white top striped with gold Lurex. She had an elegant scarf around her shoulders, but her hair was unkempt. She told me her life story. Born in Yorkshire, she worked as a bank clerk, and ended up marrying the manager. He was sixty, coming up for retirement, and she was forty. The highlight of her life, she said, was the birth of her son when she was forty-one. She had a nice house, and she loved visiting London and attending concerts – Beethoven, Chopin and Tchaikovsky were her favourites. She kept interrupting herself to apologize for boring me and for taking up my time. There was a wonderful gentility to her manner. Her wrists were as thin as broom handles and her skin was like transparent paper, so fragile that it might tear at any moment. We talked for half an hour. I noticed she had small chips of nail polish and offered to do her nails, but again she said she didn't want to take up my time.

Frank was in his room, watching a large television, but his face lit up at the idea of company. He had a big smile but it didn't match his words: no one came to visit him, everyone had forgotten him, he told me. When I expressed sympathy, he was stoical: 'That's life, isn't it? There's nothing left for me. Nothing left to me.'

His big blue eyes seemed to be searching for something. On the wall were photos of his children. They all lived locally, but none of them came to visit him, he repeated. Pride of place was a large photograph in a gilt frame of him with his wife at a wedding. Both had nosegays in their lapels. 'She kept me in order. She died beside me in the bed, ten years ago. There was no point to anything after that.'

He did thirty years in the police force, in traffic; it was better in the past – everything was better in the past. Now all he did was watch TV. 'That's all I'm good for.' When I commented on some photos of a lovely baby, he brightened. He had five grandchildren. He loved the baby and saw him often. Two of his grandchildren had got degrees, he told me proudly. His claim that he had no visitors didn't make sense. As soon as I thought I understood something of his life, the pieces fell apart again. He kept smiling his broad, heartfelt smile.

In the next room, Jacques lay on his bed in the bare room. There was a strong smell of urine. He said he felt terrible. 'It's awful here.' He wanted to talk about his family. They all lived in the same street. None of them spoke English. They spoke so many languages, he didn't know what he was supposed to speak.

'My grandparents had come from White Russia/Poland. They spoke Polish, Russian, Lithuanian, and Yiddish.'

Then he launched into a complicated explanation, raising himself from his pillow as he talked with great animation about the quarrels that had dominated his extended family. He was enjoying talking, and circled around the same questions. 'It was complicated,' he kept repeating, as he described feuds which predated the Second World War. Did the grandfather have an affair with his wife's sister? 'Absolutely not, but the aunts put that rumour around,' he replied to himself.

There were marriage breakdowns, rumours about the parentage of various children. He hadn't married himself or had any children. 'I couldn't,' he said, and launched into an explanation that never arrived. 'It was more complicated that you can ever imagine,' he added. He was as confused as he had been as a child, still struggling after all these years to make sense of his family: who was what to whom; who was a good woman and who was not. He promised to tell me more the next time I came.

Other research tasks and responsibilities intervened, and I never went back. I had a nagging sense of guilt over my promises to return. Several were people who had already been abandoned, not least by their own competent, cognitive selves. I had retreated, overwhelmed by the sheer scale of human need bursting out of that neat building. The calm orderliness underlined the routine nature of this suffering. There are thousands of similar homes all over the country. There was no outrage to be generated here, which might usefully distract one from this tsunami of need for companionship, for relationship, for laughter and life; above all, for consolation for the multiple losses of human capability – ease of movement, agency, memory, comprehension. Not to mention the loss of loved ones – the husbands, wives and mothers who had once made life meaningful. Despite finding the stories and characters fascinating, I found the care home exhausting. It felt as if the air was sucked out of me – like putting my mouth over a hoover nozzle. The only other option appeared to be to adopt the distant, bland competence used by the staff, with varying degrees of cheerfulness.

'Anguish has its own time-scale. What separates the anguished person from the unanguished is a barrier of time; a barrier which intimidates the imagination of the latter,' writes John Berger. Quoting the psychologist G. M. Carstairs, he continues: 'to encounter a fellow human being in a state of despair compels one to share, at least in the imagination, his [sic] elemental problems: is there any meaning in life? Is there any point in his staying alive?'

*

The next project I volunteered for visited people in their own homes. Gladys was in her late eighties and had severe dementia. She was being cared for by her children, with other members of the family frequent visitors; many more, in framed photos on the wall, looked down on us. The only person Gladys recognized was her deceased husband. She remembered the names of her children most of the time, but had lost track of her grandchildren, let alone her great-grandchildren. A label beside her told her what day it was, and she would ask me repeatedly what the time was. Knowledge of the world had shrunk to two names – her own and the name of her street. Every visit, she would ask me repeatedly what my name was, and where I came from; did I live here? Was I a daughter? No, and no, I said. 'Shame,' she replied, 'I love you.'

Comprehension may have been scarce – the world a place of shadows – but there were many things holding strong in Gladys: the warmth of her heart, her appetite for sweet biscuits, her humour and her sense of rhyme. She liked the sound of my name and rhymed it with one of hers – 'We're near neighbours,' she exclaimed with great delight every week. She liked the sound of my mother's name and rhymed it with a Caribbean ice-cream brand – again to peals of delight.

She caught hold of one of my fingers. 'What's this?'

My finger, I replied.

'I was going to eat it. I thought it was a sweet.'

We both laughed. She repeated wickedly, 'I was going to eat it.'

I could not bring biscuits, because she was diabetic, but she lavished love on me: 'You are like a daughter,' she insisted, and told me to tell each member of my family, 'God bless.' She repeated countless times every week, 'I love you, I love you.'

She was a reminder that loss of cognition and historical identity does not mean the loss of a 'relational self'. Dementia does not remove personality, only distort it, and the distortions themselves can be fascinating – comic, absurd, but full of warmth. She always had a member of the family with her, and frequently called out for reassurance. Where's my daughter? Is it tea time? Sometimes, the calls went on all night, I was told. She needed help with toileting, washing and dressing. She showered endearments on her daughter, but could still demand of her: 'Who are you? Are you related to me?'

I told one daughter that her mother was a remarkable, warm-hearted woman. She looked proud and pleased: 'That's my mother.' The family offered me the chance to witness how they held true to their historic knowledge of their mother. They had an understanding of dignity and courtesy and how that ordered the relations of the household; I was always introduced to new members of the family, and they made a point of seeing me to the front door every time, regardless of whatever else was happening.

On one of my visits, the geriatrician arrived. He was explaining Gladys' condition and the options for medication. He spoke in a blizzard of medical terms, at the end of which he got to his feet, smiling, and headed off, seemingly unaware of the confusion he was leaving in his wake. Sensibly, the daughter had recorded all of it on a phone, so that she could go back through it. She was tired – her mother had been awake most of the night – but there was no question of a care home. Her sense of duty was clear.

In the international bestseller *Being Mortal*, Atul Gawande writes that towards the end of life, 'the battle is to maintain the integrity of one's life – to avoid becoming so diminished and dissipated or subjugated, that who you are becomes disconnected from who you were.' His wise insight doesn't go far enough; beyond the point he describes, there may lie another struggle, where there is a disconnection between the past and the present identity, almost complete rupture. It's a place of modern-day nightmares, because we invest huge significance in our sense of self and in our identity as autonomous and independent. But in my weekly visits to Gladys over several months, I saw how her family continually reminded her of her place in the world. Deeply religious, they were supported by their belief structure and a wider community which found value and dignity in the task. I was overwhelmed by their generosity of spirit, which could find the patience and dedication over years to support not just their mother's body but her entire identity.

(vi)

dependence

dependence, noun – 1. The state of relying on or being
controlled by someone or something else. 2. Reliance; trust;
confidence.

No other mammal has such an extended period of dependence
as the human species. Foals are on their legs within hours, but
babies are entirely dependent on their carers for several years.
The human nervous system takes twenty years to develop,
while our cognitive capacities take sixteen years, compared to
eight years in a chimpanzee. The evolutionary advantage of this
long maturation is the growth of a bigger brain; co-operation
became essential in the earliest human societies to protect the
dependent young and those caring for them. Human beings
have been managing dependence for millennia through the
strong social structures of family and community. Our lives are
bookended by dependence: a long maturation to adulthood and,
now, often, a long old age.

Women and children were known as 'dependants' (although
the reality was that men were usually just as dependent on their
wives – particularly for food). Dependence has historically been
feminized and associated with weakness, but in fact dependence was also a marker of status; up to the twentieth century, the
middle and upper classes often couldn't even dress themselves,

let alone cook or bring up their children. The philosopher of care Eve Feder Kittay suggests that 'our own dependency and the dependency of others has been conveniently kept out of sight, tucked away metaphorically, and literally attended to by women'.

The second half of the twentieth century promoted a novel ideal: dependence had always been shameful for men, and increasingly it became shameful for women too; the periods of the life course when dependence was unavoidable (childhood, disability, sickness and old age) became problematic, because they did not fit the dominant narrative. Feder Kittay continues, 'as women seek to be equals, hidden dependencies become visible. Women cannot leave the home for the marketplace and abandon dependants in the process. Attempting to be in both places at once is either impossible or achieved with strain and struggle. Something gets lost, either some of the woman's autonomy and ability to compete as an equal or else the care and well-being of dependants.'

In the 1960s teenagers, eager to join this narrative, insisted on independence. In the 1980s the predominantly cultural emphasis on independence was translated into political and economic terms; in the sharp dislocation caused by deindustrialization in the 1980s and 1990s, people were expected to make their own way. The welfare state, designed to care for those periods of dependence such as old age and illness, was recast into a coercive framework to reduce it to its shortest possible time period. Independence became the culturally privileged goal, and its absence prompted contempt. The shift was deeply jarring to many aspects of social relationships, particularly as it has coincided with an ageing society. Dependency is 'a dirty word' in our society, writes the GP Jonathan Tomlinson on his blog; he admits that for a long time he has wanted to write about the 'importance and value of dependency', with help from his father, a retired vicar. Fearful of the likely response on Twitter, he had been deterred. 'Trying to mount a defence of dependence is to invite ridicule and scorn, smacks of medical paternalism.'

Maggie Kuhn, the activist and founder of the Grey Panthers movement in the US, argues for the concept's rehabilitation: 'I have learned not to feel diminished by asking for help, instead I feel a new kind of reward from human love.' When the writer and theologian Henri Nouwen was involved in a car accident and his life hung in the balance, he realized how 'life is lived from dependence to dependence', and 'my deepest being was as a dependent being'. As he waited for surgery, he 'experienced complete dependence and this experience was so real, so basic and so all pervasive that it changed radically my sense of self'.

Beatrice Webb, the pioneering advocate of state provision of welfare, was researching the living conditions of London's poor in the 1880s when her father had a stroke. As an unmarried daughter, she was required to care for him. 'I shall look back on these days here, the peace and restfulness [and] his loving dependence on me – the quiet thought and reading – with a sad regret. It has been one of the resting places of life – and so far and few between in this constant and painful struggle. It is sad watching the slow decay. My life is a perfectly dutiful life, with the sweetness of self-devotion to another whom I have loved and love still.' But such sentiments contrast strikingly with her growing frustration that she could not dedicate herself to her work, and after her father's death, she wrote in her diary that never again would she allow anyone to become dependent on her and prevent her working. She married Sydney Webb, but they had no children; she was a rare woman of her day to reject the convention that a woman's life should be entirely dominated by the dependence of others.

Questions of dependence and care are central in *King Lear*, the Shakespeare scholar Edward Wilson Lee explained to me.

'The play is shot through with reflections on care: who cares for whom? What are we entitled to expect from a caregiver? What are our obligations to our parents and to ourselves? The play explores a recurrent theme of care-lessness. The subplots rein-force the centrality of care: Edgar disguises himself to care for his father, the Duke of Gloucester, while the Duke of Kent cares for Lear when he goes mad. It is the experience of dependence and vulnerability which proves an epiphany for Lear as he dis-covers his own humanity in concern for the insane Tom when they are both wandering as outcasts on the heath.

> *'Poor naked wretches, whereso'er you are,*
> *That bide the pelting of this pitiless storm,*
> *How shall your houseless heads and unfed sides,*
> *Your loop'd and window'd raggedness, defend you*
> *From seasons such as these? O, I have ta'en*
> *Too little care of this!*

'Shakespeare's own father had died and he was the father of daughters so these questions were very personal. What obli-gations do we have to look after people who can't look after themselves? The two who survive with their moral integrity intact, Edgar and Kent, were the ones to offer care at great per-sonal risk.' Wilson Lee concludes that the word 'care' appears throughout the play in its many guises – as attention, ethical imperative, burden and responsibility.

Dependence is entered into with great reluctance and unwill-ingness; many cite it as the greatest fear of growing old. King Lear chose dependence on his two daughters and was savagely betrayed. It necessitates huge trust. Intriguingly, Buddhist monasticism explicitly requires dependence; as part of their monastic vows, nuns and monks undertake not to have or handle money, not to take anything themselves without it being explicitly offered – even details as basic as a chair or food. The monastics have to be served their food, they have to be driven, and they have to be accompanied on any journey involving money. Their monasteries are entirely dependent on donations for everything; at one Buddhist monastery in Hertfordshire, Amaravati, a noticeboard lists current shortages, such as loo paper or soap. If the gifts don't materialize, they have to do without. The Buddha's intention was that his monastic communities would always be dependent on the laity, and would thus have to find ways to serve them rather than becoming independent institutions of power. When faithfully practised, Abbot Amaro of Amaravati suggests, it is a radical way of living, a constant reminder of the reality of interdependence and a persistent humbling of the self.

7

The Ferryman's Task

AT THE DEATHBED

'Before us great Death Stands
Our fate held close within his quiet hands.'

'Death', Rainer Maria Rilke, *Poems*, 1918

The camera stayed steady on the hunched back of the oarsman as he rowed. The sides of the boat framed the shot. The viewer's vantage point was that of a prone corpse on its last journey down the Thames to the burial grounds. The soft swish of the prow cutting through the water, the steady rhythm of dipping oars, and the creaking of the boat's timbers in a journey made of sounds. Beyond the ferryman's shoulders there was only a glimpse of the sky's shifting clouds. Charon, the ferryman, took the dead across the river Styx to Hades, the kingdom of the dead. The film was short, perhaps no more than fifteen minutes, and forced us to dwell on the unimaginable: the last journey we take.

It brought back memories of sitting by my father's deathbed

as he lay in a coma, and my sense of being surplus after the weeks of trying to offer care. He had gone beyond anything I could do. The whispering in his ear or holding of his hand was now irrelevant. The film summoned another memory of being present as a relative died, surrounded by family listening intently to each of her heavy, faltering breaths until they stopped. The stillness and the silence. She had reached the other side and was at peace, finally.

No journey is as demanding, or makes its way through territory as foreign, as dying. Everyone comes to this point in life as a novice, and has to find the navigation skills needed there for the pain, grief and fear. The social anthropologist Robert Murphy likened his diagnosis of a disease of the spinal cord to a kind of 'extended anthropological field trip', in which he travelled in a 'social world no less strange to me at first than those of the Amazon forests'. He applied the same intense curiosity to the experience as he had once brought to his research in the Amazon. Writers reach for spatial metaphors to describe the alien, unfamiliar experience of serious illness and dying. Susan Sontag suggested we are all born with two passports, one to the kingdom of the well and the other to the kingdom of the sick, and at some point we emigrate. To follow the metaphor, we arrive at our sickbed and, later, our deathbed as immigrants: disorientated, homesick and unable to speak the language. From time to time, these immigrants write letters home to those still living in the kingdom of the well. In a series of columns in the *British Medical Journal*, Kieran Sweeney, a doctor, reflected on his experience of terminal illness: 'One's guides in this world have a dual role: to read the map and direct you accordingly, but also to be with you on the terrain, a place of great uncertainty'.

The ferryman needs to know how to row, how to navigate the currents of the river and where to take the passenger. We each face death alone, but generally we arrive at that point dependent on the care of others. Anyone can suddenly be called to the task of ferryman, to take up the oars, and, in however small a way, become part of the journey. Dying is a social experience, and many of us are drawn in, however reluctantly. Dying cannot be left to healthcare professionals, because it is not just a medical process. The ferryman role takes many guises, from the bringing of basic comfort and relief from suffering, the sustaining of life – laughter, friendship, pleasure – and the meanings possible on the journey, to the task of witnessing, and sharing the loss and many farewells.

Of the many forms of care investigated in this book, attending to the needs of the dying can be the most demanding – often laden with grief, and always confronting the caregivers with the foreign country of their own mortality, a place of great and usually unacknowledged fear. Interviews with those attending death had a very particular flavour: intense and exhausting, yes, but also exhilarating in their searching honesty. Here were people who had accompanied others to the edge of human experience, and were often still struggling to make sense of it.

My father had a heart attack at the age of seventy-four, three weeks after my youngest child was born. A few weeks later, we were told that all his vital organs were failing – liver, kidneys and heart – and he had only months to live. The time that followed has become an exhausted jumble of memories, in which the vulnerabilities of my baby and father were juxtaposed. I sat at his hospital bedside while an aunt pushed my screaming baby around the car park. I tried to persuade my tetchy father to eat before rushing back to breastfeed a hungry baby. Later, when my father was back home, he sat in his armchair, his shrunken form disturbingly unfamiliar. As he declined, my baby was strengthening, plump and rosy. Once fed, the baby slept deeply, utter contentment on his peaceful face, and my father was fascinated; he couldn't take his eyes off the fattening baby he called 'Jumbo', and he expressed deep envy. I've wondered since what prompted his comments: whether it was the idea of a life starting anew, the peaceful ease, or the sense of being cared for.

I was confronted with the two pivotal experiences in the life course when care is required: birth and death. They share certain characteristics: both are urgent, and can be overwhelming in their demands. They require a giving of the self without clear reciprocity: the care of the other must be the priority, and the cost can be steep – in sleep, time and freedom. Caught between these two generations, the arc of life was poignantly evident; I nurtured my baby's new capabilities while my father adjusted to their loss. As my son kicked his limbs, and strengthened his neck, my father grew frail, losing his capacity to walk or move unaided.

For those final three months of my father's life, I bounced like a ping-pong ball between the demands of a new baby and two young children and trying to support my father alongside my siblings. While I was now relatively confident as a mother, the idea of caring for my father was deeply unfamiliar. Fiercely independent, suspicious of all forms of medical care, a man of formidable determination, he was a difficult patient, full of frustration at his rebellious body. For him, the kingdom of the sick was a place of violent revolution, as the willpower that had carried him through a lifetime was rudely overthrown. What might care mean in the context of such irascible fury? I asked myself, racking the foggy remains of my sleep-deprived brain on the train north to his hospital, the baby at my breast.

On my first visit, I took him a present of a book of poetry. I had never read poetry with my father before, but I had some unconscious fantasy that, finally, we would enjoy the pleasure of reading Dylan Thomas together and find some quiet companionship at the hospital bed. Instead, he complained about the food, and I eventually inherited the book, unopened. It didn't get easier. Whenever I sat with him in those last weeks, I wondered what I was supposed to do: talk? But if so, about what? Pray? (He was a devout Catholic.) Just sit there? We tried all three, but I am not sure any of them were much help. With admirable honesty, he told me that 'dying was boring'. Nothing better summed up this man of huge appetites, whose gusto for life – for his art, love of North Yorkshire, books, friends, food and drink – had arrived at this inexplicable halt. Perhaps I could have responded that my attempt at care – these visits of confused solidarity and duty – could also be described as boring, but, looking back, I am glad of every moment I managed to sit by my father's bedside. It was an experience I needed, a closure to our relationship which has served me well in the fifteen years since. I went from listless hours at the hospice to a home teeming with the requirements of three small children, every minute packed with the labour of care – the washing, cooking, clearing up, sock sorting, and shepherding of small bodies.

Birth and death usher in dramatic new realities – a beginning or an end – and the role of midwife is needed in both. But while births prompt a plethora of advice from multiple directions, the care of the dying takes you into a quiet world. People are reluctant to describe the nature of the task, hiding behind stock phrases. Even friends honest about every other aspect of their life, were uncharacteristically terse; I didn't know if they were protecting me or themselves. One friend described caring for a close relative as akin to being in the trenches of the First World War. He didn't explain the analogy, and I didn't feel I could ask; it was rather like the war veterans who didn't want to talk about their experiences and whose families didn't like to press. I was left to assume it was one terrifying, horrifying experience after another. Equally, when I have been close to someone dying, I haven't found anyone who wanted to hear about this complicated, powerful experience; they offered a sympathetic hug, but less often a listening ear. Was it the busyness of friends, who feared that such a conversation had no easy exit point, or fear of the demanding, unfamiliar subject?

For these reasons, of all my labours of care, this is one I've had the least opportunity to discuss. It is also one of the hardest to describe, because it is riddled with paradoxes: the weight and enormity of the end of a life can be incongruously bundled together with the absurd and banal. This care entangles us like no other, bringing to the surface our relationship with the person dying and our own mortality, in a powerful constellation. Yet this intense experience, with its periods of waiting and uncertainty, is swept away by the event of death itself – the arrangements, rituals and the loss. The months or weeks of dying can often be obscured.

The doctors and nurses who work in end-of-life care admitted in interviews that they were discreet about aspects of their work. 'We edit our conversation,' a senior palliative nurse told me, acknowledging that the work could often be 'messy'. Dying is painful enough, without charting the humiliating processes by which we lose control of our bodies and discover those further reaches of dependence and vulnerability. Here, the materiality of our flesh rebels against the social conventions by which it has been disciplined during adult life, and we encounter the powerful, unforgettable smell of dying. A culture saturated by images of the idealized body – youthful, svelte, fit, lightly tanned, sexual – has banished knowledge of how the body ages, decays and disintegrates.

The discretion characterizes even the academic literature, as anthropologist Julia Lawton acknowledges. Commenting on her research in a hospice, she wrote of 'the stench of incontinence, lethargy and despondence of patients, many of whom had struggled with illness for years ... the burnout and exhaustion experienced by their family and friends. These were a far cry from the hospice literature. The protracted period of suffering that can occur prior to death is rarely if ever portrayed.' It is comforting to imagine that the end of life can be a peaceful and dignified affair, concluded Lawton, but it may not be accurate: 'romanticised images of death and dying prevalent within society can be helpful and reassuring to many people, [but] they can also lead to false expectations and to a sense of disappointment and disillusionment'. She pondered on whether this was why people often approached her after talks, wanting to discuss how they felt they had failed in their care of someone dying.

Most arrive at this task of ferryman profoundly inexperienced and unprepared. In past centuries, most adults had been present at several deaths; now it is common to reach old age without ever having seen a corpse. The medieval texts of *Ars moriendi*, 'The Art of Dying', provided advice for a good death, advocating stoicism and repentance, but there is no such consensus nowadays. Shock and bewilderment have become characteristics of the task. Listen to those who have been intimately involved in the care of a dying person and the horror reverberates through the conversation. 'Unimaginable' was how one man summed up the experience of caring for his wife, whom he had shared his life with since he was a teenager.

We may not find the words, but the ferryman does not forget the feel of the oars in their hands, the resistance of the water. Care of the dying sticks in the memory. While I remember little of the years of nappies and small toddlers, the details of the dying I have been present at, or known about, are still clear. This is where care becomes an exacting form of education, however reluctant we are to learn. In his book on his father's death, the writer Kevin Toolis concluded that 'the only way to take the weight of my own mortality was through offering to take the weight of others'.

Doctors and nurses offered me vivid stories of patients' deaths that had stayed with them, sometimes for decades, not because of their medical significance, but because of deeply moving encounters with extraordinary courage, touching warmth and deep gratitude, as well as fear. On several occasions, they were in tears as they spoke to me about moments that had inspired and shaped their understanding of their work. Care of the dying can count as one of the most powerful and lasting experiences of a lifetime, I was told more than once, and the memory is not forgotten because we know instinctively that we will need this vital knowledge of a place where we will end up in time.

Liz cared for her husband after he was diagnosed with motor neurone disease.

'Some people find it too painful to be with someone and watch the deterioration, but Oliver told me, "You have to die some day and I'm not in pain. I married the right person." My husband was six-foot-four and twice my weight. He began to fall, and I couldn't lift him. A few times ambulance staff had to come and help get him up and seated again. You had to keep your head together. We got a carer to help. A Nigerian lady in her fifties came in the morning to help wash and dress him, give him breakfast and his medication. While she did that, I could do the project management. There was so much to change and adapt in the flat; we had to find a hospital bed, and we had to chuck out a third of our furniture and half our papers to make room for all the equipment he needed. You can't imagine the amount of work. I never thought I could do it, but I did.

'I have no idea what care means – the word has been hollowed out. My mother and my sister did the carey type of thing. I worked all my life in IT, and mostly with men. My sister does the clucking bit. I love her and I see she has all the skills, but she drives me bonkers. I do things according to a plan and get it done.'

Liz had been a scientist, she reminded me, and her life was dominated by her career until she reached her fifties. She had decided against having children. 'I suppose the caring started at fifty for me; I had never done it before. I tried to support my parents. My father looked after my mother for five years after she had a stroke at eighty-one. After her death, my father lived for another five years and, shortly after his death, my husband developed *myasthenia gravis*, a muscular weakness. Four years later he was diagnosed with motor neurone disease. I told him that I wasn't much good at caring. He replied, "Then you'd better get good at it." He was in charge of his life to the very end; he used to say he was not a parcel. He was a truly astonishing man. He was complete in himself, and he knew who he was. We'd been married for forty years; there was no *I*, just *we*, we knew each other so well.

'It was a great shock to go from being very busy to this slow stream of life. Oliver was very accepting of what was happening to him, and was peaceful in his mind; there was no fear. I wouldn't say he suffered. I knew what he wanted: calm. He didn't want panic or alarm, and he certainly didn't want any drama. I knew what I had to do: don't make a mess, keep things balanced and organized.

'I was on a train in an empty carriage a short while after his death, and a woman came up to me holding something out in her hand. "It's a pearl, it's a pearl," she said, and told me that it was the first time she had been out since her husband died, and this was the third pearl she had found. Her husband had loved to give her pearls, she explained. I smiled; there wasn't really anything to say. It's the thinness of the membrane between the worlds.

'At Oliver's funeral, a crow appeared. Shortly after, it was Christmas and I was having a terrible time. I noticed a crow at the gate, looking anxiously around. It was never normally there and the message came through clearly: Pull yourself together, you're not on your own.

'I've never liked crows, but now they matter to me.

'After my mother died, my father asked me if he had cared for her well enough, and I told him that it had been the greatest achievement of his life. I think it was the greatest achievement of mine to care for Oliver. In my family we were brought up to see people through to the end, to be stalwart. There was a quality of presence in those last years: I would call it "intelligent presence" or "comprehended presence". It was not blind or unknowing. I understood what was happening and he understood that I understood, and vice versa: that was the *we*. I feel that's still there. That's what the crows are about – when I need to be brought to my senses.'

Two artists made the experience of care the subject of their work. Philip Roth looked after his father as he was dying from a brain tumour, and wrote the autobiographical memoir *Patrimony*, while the painter Paula Rego portrayed the care of her husband suffering from multiple sclerosis. Their work dates from the late 1980s and breaks through conventions surrounding dignity and privacy to a new honesty; they share an unflinching focus on the diseased body and how it destroys masculinity as independent, virile and powerful.

Roth's father was a vivid, opinionated, argumentative self-made man. Already widowed when he was taken ill, his son assumed the role of carer. So unfamiliar was this territory that it was not Roth, the wordsmith, who named his role, but his father, who confessed on the phone to a friend, 'Phillip is like a mother to me.' Little had prepared Roth for the task, but his affection for his indomitable father overrode the lack of experience or confidence. At first, it was relatively straightforward for a man with his connections: he talked to the doctors and found second opinions. At other moments he was less confident; when should he explain to his father the diagnosis, and could his father continue to live alone? He found himself unable to sleep at night, worrying.

Care is not a word Roth uses – he never referred to himself as a carer – but while the son might fight shy of the term, his father had no such inhibitions. In a letter, Roth senior defended his habit of criticising and offering advice to a grandson: 'there are many advisors in this world, also people who *care* and *do*', and he cited a list of ways in which he'd ensured his wife and his son had medical treatment. 'I care for people in my way,' he added, and admitted that part of that care was to nag (he calls it 'hocking') signing off the letter, 'The Hocker, Misnomer, it should be the carer, Love, Dad.'

Philip Roth describes one occasion when his father lost control of his bowels in the bathroom. He washed and towelled his father dry, dressed him in a clean bathrobe and led him to bed, before cleaning the bathroom. His ashamed father begged him not to tell anyone.

'I felt awful about his heroic hapless struggle . . . and about the shame of it, the disgrace he felt himself to be . . . and yet now that it was over and he was so deep in sleep I thought I couldn't have asked anything more for myself before he died. This, too, was right and as it should be.' He goes on: 'It wasn't the first time that I'd understood this either: once you sidestep disgust and ignore nausea and plunge past those phobias that are fortified like taboos, there's an awful lot of life to cherish.' Roth writes that he 'felt tenderly protective of his [father's] vulnerability', and his account of his father's actual death is sparse: 'Dying is work . . . and he was a worker.'

At much the same time as Roth was writing about his father, Paula Rego painted *The Family*, which depicts a man disabled by disease being dressed by two women. One of the carers stands on the bed behind him, her face fixed in a vague, cheerful smile, her hair in a pink bow, like a flag flying bravely from a mast. She grips the man's wrist with one hand and her other arm is across the man's face – he is at risk of being smothered in the struggle to prop him up. Clearly distressed, only one eye and a part of his forehead is visible. Another woman braces her body to pull up the father's trousers. The strain and effort is visible in the daughter's face and the eiderdown slipping off the bed. His legs jut out uselessly.

The man wears a suit and tie, an indication of his lost authority and status, but in this bedroom, he is as ungainly as a Guy Fawkes stuffed with straw, surrounded by women and the femininity of eiderdowns, red tablecloths and pink carpets. Each of the three women expresses a complicated ambivalence: frustration, even anger, as well as routine stoicism. Care is not idealized; it is not even tender, but it is brave. In the corner of the bedroom, an oratory is painted with the images of St Joan of Arc and St George, both martial saints celebrated for their courage and strength, their lives dominated by conflict and violence.

Ten years later, Rego returned to the representation of care in another painting, *The Shipwreck*. A woman sits on a sofa with a man, twice her size, spread across her lap. His eyes are closed – perhaps sleeping – as she stares to the side. She cannot move from under the weight; the position of the two figures is implausible. She could never have lifted him on to her lap – somehow he has landed on her, a reminder of the chance, unexpected nature of a cruel disease. He is half naked, as if in bed, his head is propped on a pillow: she has temporarily become his bed. His hands are crossed on his stomach, prayerful, in a gesture associated with old women. His legs hang limp, useless. It is an image of impotent masculinity, dependent on an ambivalent woman. She is wearing high heels, hinting at a life outside the sick room, and impractical for the work of caring. Her legs are braced wide, pigeon-toed, to carry the weight of him, her arm and hand strain to hold him, to stop him rolling off her knees. In the foreground, a startled animal, a skinny cat, screeches, staring fiercely straight at the viewer.

It is not just the amateurs who arrive shocked and inexperienced at the task of ferryman; many of the professionals are deeply troubled by how we care for the dying, and by what they are expected to offer. Intrusive procedures such as resuscitation and feeding by tube needlessly prolong life and suffering, argues consultant Seamus O'Mahony in his disturbing book *How We Die*, and he suggests that the treatment of the dying is 'notable not for kindness but for cowardice, evasion and humbug'. The urgency of this critique is also evident in Atul Gawande's *Being Mortal*; death and old age have been medicalized, he writes, in an 'experiment in social engineering' which has failed.

Gilly, a senior nurse in Accident and Emergency, was deeply distressed in her interview with me: 'No one is allowed to die now, so even old ladies are brought in from nursing homes and the doctors will try to resuscitate them, and then they die anyway.' She was emphatic: 'The last hours of someone's life should not be in A & E. We invariably have drunks here and all sorts going on. They need dignity and reverence. It's one of the things I have great issue with.'

Another nurse I shadowed on the wards admitted she was also uncomfortable: 'It is not uncommon on a busy ward for someone to die alone. The other day a patient was admitted and died half an hour later. The family didn't want to come in, and he died on his own. I was busy on another job. It happens,' she said grimly, and then added bleakly, 'Some days you go home and cry.'

Most deaths are in hospitals and yet most people say they would prefer to die at home. Much of the recent debate on dying has been dominated by questions of choice and efforts to establish a 'preferred place of death'. Dr Caroline Nicholson, a palliative-care consultant nurse, is infuriated by the meaninglessness of the rhetoric: 'Why does this issue of where you die dominate? I'll tell you – because it's measurable, and it plays into questions of "choice". But it's lazy, and doesn't think about all the variables which affect place of death. It sounds simple, but it isn't. To suggest there is a choice pushes demands back on to the NHS and social care for which there are no resources. Giving people "a choice" when one doesn't know what the choice consists of, or when there isn't one, is one of the most hideous forms of covert manipulation. Yet it sounds benign: who can deny that a dying person should choose where to die? It becomes difficult to shine the light on this without sounding cynical, or as if you don't want this as an aim, but the real issues when you are dying are about citizenship, feeling held and loved. Things often have to be negotiated and flexed, and the question is whether there is a "holding community" for the dying person. That's a "good enough" death, and we are in danger of losing this capacity.'

Most people die in busy wards where staff have little time and sometimes little training to offer support. Despite the popularity of hospices, only 40 per cent of the dying and their carers use their services. The last year of life entails, on average, nearly three emergency admissions, a total of around 1.5 million in England each year. The costs of such treatment are rising, and there is widespread agreement that more appropriate services for the dying are urgently needed. Many relatives are left deeply unhappy by their experience of a death in an acute hospital, citing the impersonality, lack of sensitivity and dignity; over half of complaints to the NHS relate to the care of the dying. Scientific medicine and healthcare systems are designed to cure disease and fix injury; death is seen as a form of failure. We have ended up with this most private and personal of experiences happening in institutions with inappropriate agendas of acute medical care and efficiency.

Half a million people die every year in England and Wales, and for three quarters of them, it is a protracted process. How we die has changed: it is rarely sudden or quick, unlike in the past. Most of the dying are very old, and have had an extended period of frailty and vulnerability, lasting six years on average. A growing proportion of this group are suffering from dementia, which will affect one in three of those over eighty-five. Many in this age group have multiple chronic conditions requiring complex routines of medication and care and recurrent visits to hospital as they slowly become more frail. Modern medicine has made dying a long process full of small advances and bigger setbacks; it can be exhausting for all concerned – both the person dying and those attempting to offer support.

This pattern of slow dying cannot be fitted into any of the institutional healthcare structures developed in the UK. It falls between the gaps of a health system designed around acute care. Extensive lobbying by the hospice movement and charities in recent years has had only limited success in improving the community services needed. At the point of our greatest vulnerability, there can be little help available; we are suddenly and unexpectedly thrown back on the resources of family, friends and often, our own finances.

'The huge elephant in the room is this combination of three things: the state doesn't provide care, people are living for longer, and the family is too attenuated to care,' commented Nicholson. 'We split people into the living and the dying, but the frail elderly are doing both, and our medical system doesn't allow for that. My life's work is about putting these two back together, so that we grasp how we live and die at the same time. Prognostication has become the holy grail, but what is much more complex and unknown is this parallel process of people living and dying over time.'

Nicholson's PhD followed the cases of frail elderly people

over a period of seventeen months. In one distressing case, she recalls, an elderly man was disintegrating both mentally and physically. The family couldn't cope and looked for help. 'He went to hospital, but they said they couldn't do any more for him and sent him home. He was bouncing in and out of hospital. The palliative-care teams wouldn't see him, because there were no symptoms for them to manage. Many of our multidisciplinary meetings in the hospice are about sick people whose carers can no longer cope, but the person is deemed not sick enough to justify a night sitter. We have a gentleman at the moment and we are thinking of giving him sedation at night to help him stay at home. If he fell at night, he's likely to fracture a hip and end up in A & E.'

Caring for the dying has not just become medicalized, it has also been bureaucratized. Time is central to how care is rationed. Hospices have criteria about when they will offer care and how long for. One of bureaucracy's defining features is its insistence on predictability, but death is notoriously unruly. A terminal prognosis should never include dates, declared a consultant in palliative care. Despite her experience, she often got the issue of timing wrong. The US insurance industry has invested in considerable research to predict the moment of death in order to ease the bureaucratic process of paying out health costs – with little success. Carers can find themselves grappling with an absurdity: namely, how to fit death neatly into a timetable.

The criteria used to apportion end-of-life care are complex, explained Pete, the community nurse mentioned in Chapter 4, when I shadowed him on his round of home visits. As we drove along the country lanes, I tried to keep track of the acronyms and criteria for care. The application for funding for end-of-life care had to be made directly to the UK Department of Health, and the form ran to fifty-four pages, he explained. It could take seven months or more to be granted, and was often rejected on a technicality. Some people (or their carers) ended up suing the NHS to get the care – if they had time. Another funding stream required the patient to be in the last twelve weeks of life. Pete commented wryly that by the time this book is published, the system will have changed again.

On the day I spent with Pete, he had to brief six NHS care workers who were assigned to make daily visits to Mike, an elderly gentleman with motor neurone disease. Pete had to explain to them the likely last stages of Mike's life. The care workers were on a rota to dress, feed and wash him in the home he shared with his wife. Most had now known the couple for nearly a year, and had seen his painful decline. Earlier, I had been with Pete on his visit to Mike; he was losing control of his limbs and could no longer speak, but he understood the conversation, and when he wanted to intervene, he put out his hand. Sometimes he took a notepad and wrote in shaky letters, one on top of another. He made a thumbs-up gesture when someone guessed his meaning, and with great effort would raise his head and smile.

The care workers sat around the large meeting table in silence. They rarely came into the office, and mostly worked alone on their visits, so they didn't know each other. Pete was clear and precise about the likelihood that Mike would choke.

'You can ring 999, but they won't get there in time. You can pat him on the back five times, as you have been trained. After that, there is nothing you can do. His wife has the medication to calm him and she can administer that.'

One of the care workers started to cry. Neither of those sitting beside her made any gesture of comfort. It would be wrong to call them colleagues, and they could end up being the only healthcare worker to support the wife dealing with Mike's death. Several began to blink back tears.

'If he is coughing, that's a good sign, because it means the air is going in as well as out.' Pete paused before adding quietly, 'It is very distressing to see someone die by choking.'

The room was very quiet and one woman was crying silently, the tears rolling down her face. The care manager went around the table to put a hand on her shoulder. 'We're here to support you,' she murmured. But her comment barely registered on the care workers' faces; everyone knew it was only half true.

Mike was a tall man, and his movements were so ungainly and awkward that it was a struggle to get him up, washed and dressed, even in an hour. If the carers overran, they had a race to their next call. Pete and the manager ended the session by saying how grateful they were for their work, but the faces of the support workers were blank.

On the way back to his office, Pete admitted he was concerned. 'They haven't had the training I've had. They are thrown into difficult situations repeatedly, day in, day out, with patients who have complex acute conditions. It's much easier for me. I fly in and out, but they deal with it on a daily basis. What happens if they are there at the moment of death? What support will there be for them?'

The bleakness of those support workers' faces was one of the most painful moments in all my research. Their expressions said it all: so many resources have been stripped from those who face this painful underside of life. Most obviously, they do not have the time, nor adequate financial recompense, but also they cannot lean on a shared cultural understanding of death, and they cannot expect society to acknowledge or value their part in it. Their isolation was not just from each other, but from a wider social context which could give meaning or dignity to the experience. What they were left with was the tragedy and the unmitigated rawness of physical deterioration.

On our visit, Pete had asked Mike's wife if there was someone – a friend or neighbour – she could call if she needed help.

No, she said; her son was several hours' drive away. As Pete left, Mike looked up and his face grimaced with sadness. He held Pete's hand, and tears ran down his face. He knew time was running out. He had asked when he might die and how, and had understood the answers. A brave man was frightened. Pete held his hand and patted his arm. It was all he could do.

Marion Coutts cared for her husband, the art critic Tom Lubbock, for two years before he died, aged fifty-two, from a brain tumour. Her prize-winning account of that time, *The Iceberg*, is a 'book of witness', she told me. It is a rare and vivid portrayal of care as Tom slowly lost his capacity for language and speech.

'I wrote the book because I wanted people to have the feel of it, to put into language what the experience felt like. The book is not about dying, but about living while dying, about parenting, connecting and belonging, and what happens to all this when it is under assault from the systems of health and social care. Our connection wasn't assaulted by the illness, we maintained that connection until the end.

'It depended on my paying close attention all the waking hours. That seemed to me an ethical response – to help him, but also to write about it. I felt I had to be very exact about the words and not fluff things. I wasn't the only one paying close attention – he was too. He had an intellectual enjoyment of the process, and he said as much: 'Of course I am helpless. And so what do I do with helplessness?'

'We were a young family. A decision we made was to look outward, to keep his dying social. What happened to Tom was extraordinary, improvised, exciting. Our circle of friends invented new ways to be with him when the conversation began to go, and it was fun – that was an amazing thing. It was a challenge to be with him, because it was unpredictable, and even having a conversation was full of risks.

'A lot of care comes down to attentiveness – a focused, specific attentiveness to the realm that the other is operating in, so that you are attentive to facts before they arise. Nothing else needed my attention. That felt like a positive rather than a negative. In fact it felt more important than a job, or anyone else's job. Someone said to me that this dying has been the most important part of your life, and she was right. All the stuff normally hidden on a daily basis became suddenly very clear. I felt the sense of bearing witness was instructive – if only for me.

'From the diagnosis onwards, my experience of time changed. The pressure on each individual moment changed: casual went out of the window and everything had to be deliberate. Daily life felt physically and mentally different. We all operate on the assumption that things will go on, there is always a connection to the future – the hopes, longings and plans – but for Tom, our son and me, the future was here, now. People trotted out clichés such as, "You have to live each day as it comes." I got pissed off, because taking that literally is a form of mental disorder. I didn't fantasize about alternatives. I was glued to what was happening. I became really compe-tent. It was insane, because the fields of competence required were so vast. I was always running to catch up. All the time I was thinking, learning, understanding new things about treat-ments, drugs, diseases. A super-competence took over – or at least it felt like that – fuelled by stress.

'When Tom was in hospital, I was aware of the charismatic power he had, even when he had no words. Once, I arrived early at the hospital to give him his clothes. The curtains were round his bed and three women were giving him a bed bath; they were talking in several languages. It was an amazing image to stumble on. Tom was totally relaxed. It was like a private party. I couldn't have arranged it better. I certainly couldn't have bought it. It was priceless. It was important, I felt, to bear witness to that kind of work, which is low paid and undervalued. It needs to be spoken about.

'You could feel the levels of attentiveness in staff from the way they walked, their tone of voice, their touch. One consultant was under huge pressure, but she managed to keep that hidden from us. She made us feel like she had all the time in the world for us – to manage that professionally and personally is high art. It was gobsmacking.'

As Tom's condition deteriorated, he needed more care than Marion could provide. The routines they had developed with friends to help him through the early stages of the disease were no longer adequate. The encounter at this stage with the care offered by the health service and the local authority proved traumatic.

'There was a lot of anger in the book. Our own patterns of how to live and how to care came up against other people's. You spend aeons of time waiting around in the care industry, and don't get me started on the architecture, the demoralizing power of the spatial realm of hospitals. I recognize that it was not possible to have a perfect system. People slightly danced around us, because they knew we were capable of making a fuss; it is so much harder for those who have no one to advocate for them.

'We were allocated carers who came into our home to help. One carer left our front door open, another didn't know Tom's name, and some were actively hostile. This care was imposed on us, and getting someone who was kind and responsive was a matter of chance. They had no respect for us as people or for our privacy. One of us may have been very ill, but at least we were still ourselves, and they threatened that selfhood: it was a shock. The system is completely dysfunctional in terms of low pay and training, and yet it's also expensive. This was the point where I could have unravelled. I stopped work and signed off sick.

'Luckily we only had to experience that for two and half

weeks, because Tom suddenly deteriorated and went into hospital. After five weeks, the hospital wanted us out, and that was frightening. We had been going to this hospital for nearly two and half years, and I thought I understood and knew the system, but suddenly there was no system. Tom needed twenty-four-hour medical care by this point. The hospital wanted Tom to go into a nursing home, but no home would offer medical care. We had reached an impasse – we were waiting for something to give. Hospices don't want people until they are about to die – they can offer respite care, but no more. We couldn't stay at home because there were too many stairs. We were being offered non-choices. It was very frightening, and I feared what it would be like for others, less capable of navigating the situation.

'In the end, Tom went into a hospice, where he stayed for six weeks before he died. That is a long time for a hospice, and in one meeting a doctor joked that they were not going to chuck us out. It was a terrible shock, because I hadn't understood that was an option. Where would we have gone if they had? I took comfort from the fact that once you're in, it's hard to get you out.

'The last five months could have been a fuck up, and that's frightening. Dying is bad enough. It wasn't that I expected a smooth trajectory, but my hunch is that if Tom had died in a crappy place away from us, that anger would have been really damaging for me and our son. The way it happened – in the hospice – was a form of salvation; we were given a place to be together, but I have a stark awareness of how so much of that was down to chance.

'Hospitals deprive people of their contexts – their families, connections and activities. Context was supremely important for Tom, and he was having as good a time as was possible as he was dying. The hospice understood that. They were hugely flexible. Tom's work was shown in an exhibition in the last few weeks of his life, and on the opening night the hospice assigned a nurse to accompany us. We were given a future that lasted thirty-four days, and it was vital to us; we weren't shut down. Tom was allowed to be himself in this new, shifting form. Brain cancer took his mobility and his language but not his powers of recognition; he always knew us, knew what was happening. Dying didn't take his character.'

Some professionals are passionate about how to improve end-of-life care. 'I went into palliative care because I felt that medicine had failed. The experts had taken death and made it into something abnormal,' said Dr Caroline Nicholson. 'Medicine is best when it is mediating new realities and uses interventions to help people to be in that new space, and prepare for the spaces to come. But a lot of people in palliative care don't see that as their job, so they end up making our reality feel unreal – they talk of making you feel better. I agree with symptom control, of course, but the real issue is: what are you going to use your time left for? How will you use the invitation you have been given? What fascinates me is how people negotiate that reality, and what we as a society – and me as an individual – can learn and replicate.'

This was the approach adopted by B. J. Miller, a palliative-care doctor in San Francisco and a passionate advocate on the subject. He draws on his own extraordinary life story to illustrate how he sees his work. He was electrocuted at the age of nineteen, jumping on an electric train as a prank; he was in a burns unit for a year, and lost both legs and one arm. He talks about pain and suffering with rare authority and is a compelling speaker. His online TED talk is one of its most popular downloads. Briefly in London for a conference, he found time to explain his ideas to me.

'Suffering is the single fulcrum in this field of palliative care, and you need to distinguish between necessary and unnecessary suffering. Suffering is fundamental to human experience, but we can have pain and not suffer; it's a subjective phenomenon. It flips the power dynamic of the patient-doctor relationship, because there is so much the doctor can learn from the patient – it's humbling. Suffering is a learning opportunity. It rightsizes our ego, without which we keep expanding and bloating. It's a sculpting tool.

'I can call attention to the choice of words when the patient beats themselves up for being sick, and uses the language of "fighting" and "wars": these forms of suffering are unnecessary. Part of my role is to "sanctify" grief, to acknowledge the losses of dying. The role of carer can be advocate, advisor, reflective device and sounding board. I call it a practice of "safe love".'

In an interview with the *New York Times*, Miller explained that 'Parts of me died early on in my life, and that's something, one way or another, we can all say. I got to redesign my life around this fact, and I tell you, it has been a liberation to realize you can always find a shock of beauty and meaning in what life you have left.'

After recovering from his accident, Miller switched his studies to art history. He needed to understand how to play with perspective, he explained, and by way of illustration he recounted an anecdote of a visit to a primary school, where the children asked him what it was like to have only one hand. He told them that his one hand was wonderful.

'There is a playfulness to perspective. At some point you start to focus on what you have left rather than on what you have lost.' In the aftermath of his accident, he refused to see his life as extra difficult, 'only uniquely difficult, as all lives are, sitting somewhere on a continuum between the man on his deathbed and the woman who misplaced her car keys.'

He tells the story of a wondrous instance of care which he received in the burns unit, a sterilized environment, in the basement of the New Jersey hospital. 'Burn units are houses of pain, believe me. They are not pleasant places to be or to work in, so they attract remarkable people. There were no windows, so we didn't know if it was day or night. Everyone is gowned up and there are no visitors. I knew it was snowing, because the nurses were talking about how hard it had been to drive to work. One of the nurses went out and came back with a snowball and placed it in my hand. It reacquainted my body with something which wasn't about pain, trauma and the ministrations of the nurses. That moment was so many things: the kindness of the nurse, the sensory experience of feeling something, and the wonder of it all. It had both a symbolic and a direct experiential value. It's amazing to have a body which feels all these things. It made me love life and all that was going on around me.

'I cannot tell you the rapture I felt holding the snow in my hand; the coldness dripping on to my burning skin, the miracle of it all, the fascination as I watched it melt and turn into water. In that moment, just being any part of this planet, in this universe, mattered more to me than whether I lived or died.'

After art history, he went on to study medicine. 'I fell in love with palliative care and its key principles: learning from illness, living until you die; trying not to fear death. These should be the characteristics of all care. Death is not just a clinical process, it leaves no one out: the expertise is about being human. Doctors are not the experts.

'In palliative care, we refer to "existential suffering". It's a wastebasket term. A doctor can work on the pain and depression with pills, but what is still left is the existential suffering. I see this as a crisis of meaning. I would say it's the number-one presentation in every doctor's surgery. This is huge: the somatization of isolation and meaninglessness in physical pain and all sorts of conditions.

'As a doctor, my job is to show up and be affected and accept my role in the patient's narrative-making. We have power as physicians, our patients hang on to what we say and how we act. There is so much symbolism in everything we do. Doctors have a disproportionate role in people's lives, and that's evident in palliative care. We have to be present, but presence is a dying art, because we are faced with a smorgasbord of distractions. Presence is a skill, a gift, a way of being in the world. Sometimes caring for someone can be just to accompany them – that can include awkward silences. Palliative care is essentially the act of not running away.'

Miller questions why the public debate on dying and death is dominated by the issue of choice – in particular, the two questions of when and where to die. He points out that in the countries where assisted dying has been legalized, it is used by a tiny proportion of people (4 per cent of deaths in the Netherlands). 'If assisted dying is about relieving suffering, why isn't this huge debate linked to an increased interest and investment in palliative care, which is also about relieving suffering?'

'We talk about control as if we always want it, but a) you can't always have it, and b) there are aspects of control that you wouldn't want anyway. How much can we control? We are fixated on finding, creating and maintaining control, but we have to be real about the stuff we can't control, and that's what is interesting. It puts our ego into proportion. It's a humbling truth, and in that lies knowledge and mystery.'

In *A Fortunate Life*, John Berger writes of the doctor as a 'familiar of death' – someone who has witnessed many deaths and, as such, brings confidence to the dying person and their relatives. Doctors have a value as intermediaries: they connect the dying with the 'multitudinous dead'. Berger concludes, 'the hard but real comfort which they offer is ... that of fraternity'.

Over the course of her career as a nurse in palliative care,

Jane has become such a 'familiar of death'; friends, neighbours and acquaintances instinctively turn to her when facing death.

'As a nurse, you are bearing witness to another's suffering. You are alongside them. You might not be able to do much to make things better, but you are absolutely with them. You hear what they say, and understand some of what they are feeling, and you are not running away – even though sometimes you want to, because it's awful. Very experienced nurses are almost like a mirror to people: they know when to withdraw and when to intervene. Intuitively, they create an environment for the patient and the family to do the dying. It can be very complex when someone is really suffering and the family are in conflict. It's exhausting, but it is also uplifting. These are the most powerful moments, and they are rewarding.

'This is humanity at its most intense and naked. I'm not religious, but I was brought up Catholic and my parents taught me kindness, tolerance and compassion. I have enormous belief in humanity rather than God, and that gives me great meaning in life. I have the sense that we are all in this together, we experience much the same thing. It's the basis for what I do.

'In my palliative-care work, I see really moving acts of kindness. Sometimes it's just very simple things, such as people being generous of themselves, it's not always about "doing" something. A colleague really put herself out recently to get a young patient to a football match. He had a severe illness and was very fragile, and had never been to a match. He said it had been the best day of his life. The spontaneity of this kind of generosity is really important. There is something about telling people they have to do this or that which destroys it and makes it inauthentic – and nauseating.

'The question is: how do you maintain that inner response? Compassion and care have to flourish from within. My training in the 1970s was about finding your own capacity for compassion;

you were allowed to find and develop it in your own way. I was trained by a very inspirational person. Now there is a huge emphasis on compliance and regulation. Hospices are changing – they have an identity crisis, and there is a big recruitment problem.

'Sometimes there are really practical things you can do to make people more comfortable, or to have the conversations which help them. We had a young patient with motor neurone disease recently, and he was in a lot of distress, so the nurses spent a lot of time over two days helping him to feel more comfortable. Then he asked to be taken off the breathing machine so he could talk to his family, and shortly after he died. The nurses were very proud of his peaceful death. That's what we are here for.'

Jane was emphatic that a nurse can only manage this kind of demanding work when supported by others. Care of the dying has to be a web of multiple relationships, each supporting and caring for the other. 'There was an important moment in my career when I was looking after a young man with AIDS in the late 1980s. We got on very well. He told me he was going to a hospice and he thanked me for my care on the hospital ward. He was dying –'

She stopped, choked with tears at the thirty-year-old memory.

'I had a choice: I could go to the loo and pull myself together, or I could go to one of the other nurses and tell her, I am going to cry and I need you to sit with me – that's what I did. I learnt that I needed to show these emotions, and if you don't, there is a danger of burnout. I cry a lot in my work.'

One of the most rewarding periods of her career was research she did into nurses' conversations. She was concerned that the system of SBA (Situation, Background, Action), instituted in ward handovers, had regulated how nurses shared and reflected on their work and supported each other. She and her fellow researchers argued that informal conversations were essential to the work of caring for the dying. The burden of the work is only manageable when carried collectively, they suggested. Solidarity is central – the fact that coffins are always carried by several people, often with their arms around each other's shoulders to support the weight, is a persistent tradition precisely because of its symbolism.

'Nurses are dealing with a lot of emotions and they develop rituals in their teams to cope. It could be black humour – a quick laugh in the sluice – or it could be a ritual of wanting to keep a bed empty for twenty-four hours after a death as a form of acknowledgement. They don't like the sense that they are on a conveyor belt. Without such symbols and rituals, they flounder.

'We don't talk in society about illness, dependency and death, and the people who work with these are regarded as tainted. People can't look at reality – it is too painful – so they resort to stereotypes, such as the nurse as an angel or a devil. Nurses are often dealing with awful situations. Sometimes you feel that you are in a secret society; I have never read anything which voices my experience. I've had nineteen years of ward management, but I've never heard anyone talk about what it is really like. You often feel invisible as a nurse, and low self-esteem is endemic in this job.'

Cathy, who has been a social worker in palliative care for fifteen years, shares Jane's view that care of the sick and dying is not understood. 'Care is about constant learning and that's not well understood by people. I know there is always more to learn. Every patient is new; every time it is like starting from scratch and I like the energy that generates. It's not about dragging people to where we think they should be. I had a friend who was diagnosed with cancer and I knew she was choosing to under-stand things in a certain way; some people need permission to do that. There was another individual who insisted on giving the doctor her CV. She had only four months to live and a long history of mental ill health and high levels of anxiety. But she was also an artist and she wanted to be known by more than her health problems.

'Care is very multidimensional, and every bit of communication and interaction is a process of mutual influence. A lot of caring professionals are too insular to see that the other person is influencing how they behave. I trained in systemic theory and that has helped me to step back and be curious about people's responses. I learnt a lot from Carl Rogers' work on empathy and positive regard, so that you see the person as the expert on themselves – and you always see the person. There is a process of recognition here.'

Cathy moved into palliative care after looking after her dying mother in her early thirties. 'Caring for my mother was the most exhausting thing I have ever done. I had been living abroad but I left my job and moved back to Teeside without a moment's hesitation.

'I'm interested in language and I notice that we often link care and a burden, but looking after my mother was one of the most rewarding things I've ever done. I felt I was making her investment in me worthwhile; she was a very devoted mother and had always put us children first. I knew she would have preferred me to give her a wash than someone she didn't know. She would have done the same for me. My mother was very good company. She was very witty and even when she was ill and dying, she was funny.'

In palliative care, one had to be tolerant of failure, Cathy commented, but not complacent. I wondered how this fine difference between tolerance and complacency is understood by managers, families and patients. It can take huge courage and humility to be present and tolerate some of the forms of failure

evident at death – the despair, panic, the grief, the anger and
shock. 'Sometimes I make a difference – and I'm happy with
that,' Cathy concluded.

Such modesty is an essential attribute of the 'familiar of death'.
Dying is a dramatic event which provokes intense and powerful emotion. The care I have observed and admired at the
deathbed is full of tact. Knowing how to withdraw as well as
how to give comfort, always recognizing the central roles of
others. Libby, a young consultant in palliative care, had seen
how ordinary people, not just professionals, could develop
such skills. As a twenty-two-year-old medical student on a
placement in Kerala, southern India, she worked on a project
which determined her route into becoming a palliative-care
consultant. The Kerala Neighbourhood Network in Palliative
Care trains volunteers to go into the homes of people who
are dying to offer basic pain relief and care; within ten years
of its founding the project has recruited and trained 12,000
volunteers and cares for 10,000 patients at any one time. It
helps cover the gap between inadequate hospital care for the
dying and overstretched families. The concept, now known as
Compassionate Neighbours, has won acclaim across the world
and been widely imitated.

'In Kerala I saw how the project decentralized doctors and
made death a social issue,' Libby explained. 'The community
took responsibility. It was a social movement, and the volunteers
came from all walks of life – men and women, young and old.
I saw a whole vision of what dying could be like and I knew
I wanted to set up a project based on its principles here in
the UK. Compassionate Neighbours is not about patients and
professionals, but about people as equals. It's about developing
meaningful relationships and reciprocity. The volunteers relate
to the patients as equals, travelling, sharing and holding the

suffering. There can be real intimacy. The care of the dying should be mutual and enabling. That's my central conclusion.'

Funerals are weighted with symbolism, as the bereaved assert the value of someone's life, their achievements and times of great happiness. It's a collective statement. The ritual is both for the dying person and those left behind. It's the final act of care for the person who has died, but it is also an act of care for those grieving and an expression of solidarity.

'I think you can only really die well if you leave parts of yourself continuing in those around you,' said Dr Caroline Nicholson. 'Your life has meant something and that life carries on. For the elderly, the connections with the young are the most important. In my research, I remember one elderly lady saying to me that she loved watching children running up and down the stairs. She could no longer use the stairs, let alone run, but she took pleasure from watching their freedom of movement. It was the extraordinary in the ordinary. She had this fascinating ability to find a way of leaving by identifying bits of herself in things that were continuing.'

My friend Carla's funeral was beautiful. A gregarious, warm-hearted Italian, she left behind children, husband, siblings and parents. On the day of her funeral snow lay heavily across London. As we arrived at the church, flurries greeted the coffin heaped with flowers. Pastel-coloured poppies, white blooms and trailing greenery filled the church, as if it were a wedding.

My father was in a coma for several weeks, the last life slowly ebbing out of this strong-willed, stubborn man in a silent hospice room; in dramatic contrast, his funeral was solemn, a full Catholic requiem mass at the monastery which had shaped his life from boyhood until retirement. The accounting for his life was generous, and the monks chanted the Latin plainsong which had been the anthem of his education and faith. The abbey church was full of family – those Irish Catholic roots which insist on attending funerals – and friends. His children and many grandchildren followed the coffin in a long procession. The funeral lent a grandeur to the moment; it transmuted the painful detail of his physical disintegration in a bare room in an East London hospice into an event of importance and dignity. The finality of this last act of care has repercussions for decades.

Knowing how things end, should end, can end, is a vital skill in life, perhaps even more important than knowing how they begin. My father's ending served not just him but all those present that chilly November day, as it affirmed the value and dignity of a single life. He would have appreciated his funeral. Such ritual was important to him, and in his will he asked for masses to be said. He had organized the care of his soul in the afterlife.

(vii)

suffering

Suffering, noun – The state of undergoing pain, distress, hardship, from Latin *sufferer* (as *ferre*, bear).

Suffer, verb – Experience or be subjected to (something bad or unpleasant). *Archaic*, Allow, tolerate.

'Modern medical bureaucracy and the helping professions are oriented to treat suffering as a problem of mechanical breakdown requiring a technical fix,' writes Arthur Kleinman, a psychiatrist and medical anthropologist; he suggests that suffering is 'this most thickly human dimension of patients' stories'. Clinical and behavioural-science researchers possess no category to describe suffering, he continues. 'They may quantify functional impairment with symptom scales and survey questionnaires, but on suffering, they are silent.' In contrast, medieval Christianity and Buddhism did not see 'suffering as a totally disvalued experience to be managed ... but an occasion for the work of cultural processes to transcend pain and dying.' In *Adam Bede* George Eliot referred to suffering as a 'baptism, a regeneration, the initiation into a new state'.

'Pain is a sensation and suffering is a practice,' argues the philosopher Ivan Illich; his controversial thesis was that 'the medicine which convinced people that all pain is curable, has

made pain unendurable'. He suggested that pain can be borne
with dignity by 'duty, love, fascination, routines, prayer and
compassion', but the cultural authority of medicine with its
false promises to abolish pain, suffering and death, had robbed
people in the West of their ability to suffer with dignity and
meaning. More recently, James Davies developed a similar
argument in *The Importance of Suffering*, suggesting that in contemporary understanding 'much of everyday suffering is [seen
as] a damaging encumbrance best swiftly removed'. This belief
is 'increasingly trapping us within a world view that regards all
suffering as a purely negative force in our lives', and he argues
that 'the contented life is not solely attained through rational
advancement and direct pursuit of happiness but through our
being willing to confront experience and learn from our suffering'. He quotes the Swiss philosopher Henri Frédéric Amiel:
'You desire to know the art of living, my friend? It is contained
in one phrase: make use of suffering.'

A doctor may be able to prescribe painkillers, the nurse can
administer them at the right time, but neither can necessarily
know how to respond to, or ease the existential suffering of loss.
That sense of inadequacy, of partial failure, can be heard haunting the narratives of caregivers. How they acknowledge it varies
from denial, discomfort, indifference and real distress, to anger
at the meaninglessness of the suffering. Faced with suffering, we
are left scrabbling for shared meaning which might offer some
consolation or relief, however slight.

The experience of suffering can come as a profound shock,
bringing a sense of alienation; the brain surgeon Henry Marsh
writes of the 'underworld of suffering'. It is often hidden or
ignored. Kleinman sees 'empathic witnessing' as a commitment
to the suffering person which encourages the development of a
narrative 'that will make sense of and give value to the experience'. Both caregiver and sufferer contribute to that narrative

and both have the potential to gain meaning from it. 'Moral insight can emerge from the felt experiences of sympathy and empathy,' he adds, and proposes that this is the 'inner moral meaning of chronic illness and care'.

The medical sociologist Arthur Frank asserts that generosity is central in the dilemmas provoked by suffering. Medical care 'both sets and reflects standards for caring relationships between individuals in a society', and 'by this overused word care, I mean an occasion when people discover what each can be in relationship with the other'. The role of the doctor or nurse is to offer the generosity of 'the grace to welcome those who suffer'. While medicine provides diagnoses and drugs, it should also always offer consolation, and that can amount to 'one person's promise not to abandon another' and in the process, perhaps, 'inviting some shift in belief about the point of living a life that includes suffering'.

8

Possible Futures

'Attention is the rarest and purest form of generosity.'

SIMONE WEIL,
First and Last Notebooks, 1942–3

Care is a mighty empire with many colonies, and I have only visited a few of them. My journeys have come to an end, and as I look back over the hundreds of pages of notes on people's lives, I see common patterns. In part, I have been charting the impact of austerity policies brought in by UK governments since the 2008 global financial crash, as the NHS has struggled to keep up with growing demand, and as savage cuts in social-care budgets have fallen disproportionately on people with disabilities and the elderly. More investment in the care economy is urgently needed; it is not the luxury sometimes depicted by 'small state' advocates, but essential to the social fabric and the stability and security of millions of lives. But increased funding, while essential, is not sufficient. The origins of the crisis of care predate the financial crisis of 2008 and the slashing of welfare spending which followed. The deeper cause of the crisis is a fundamental failure to value – and appropriately reward – the centrality of relationship in all care. The rhetoric is there, the policy labels are in place – personalization, person-centred care – but the reality has gone awry. Interviewees again and again lamented and demonstrated how the time and opportunities for face-to-face relationships have been progressively marginalized. The impact for both the carer and the recipient is deeply damaging, given that care is, by definition, dealing with vulnerability and dependence. Our sense of dignity rests on the actions of others; without relationship, interactions can swiftly become degrading and humiliating. Care is balanced on this fine edge because it is often dealing with the basic fragility of human lives.

This was brought home to me by a clumsy routine mammogram. The nurse was late and running behind on appointments; lines of us were waiting in a silent waiting room when she arrived. Impatiently, she hustled several of us into cubicles to undress. Then I was thrust against the machine, my flesh prodded and shoved between the plates with no more than a cursory greeting. Her focus was to get me in and out of the appointment as fast as possible. I was simply a body. What was startling was my reaction: I was shaken to the core, reduced to tears at the sudden humiliation in the dehumanizing process. I glimpsed the impact of rough treatment of the body and scanty acknowledgement of the person which can become a frequent experience for many elderly people. Unbeknown to us most of the time, our sense of dignity is precarious, resting on a set of conventions around relationships with others and the privacy of our bodies.

This vulnerability can generate powerful connection – I still remember with gratitude the tact and sensitivity of one midwife – and a deep sense of purpose and fulfilment, but it can also provoke uncomfortable emotion in both the carer and the recipient; care calls into question cherished beliefs about independence and autonomy, and always entails judging risk.

The skill of the carer lies in knowing how to contain their own emotions while remaining present, and being able to recognize the person beyond the frailty. It is a deceptively demanding task, and is a form of emotional labour which has to draw deeply on the carer's life experience and world view. It can only be sustained by strong relationships with colleagues and managers. The frequent absence of both is part of what makes home care particularly challenging.

The marginalization of relationships may be most graphic and disturbing in low-paid parts of the care economy, but it has infiltrated virtually every dimension of care. I saw all too vividly how GPs struggle through their workload, as patients pass through on a conveyor belt of appointments, each lasting a few minutes. Nurses apologize for pausing to talk to a patient, and spend a large portion of their time in front of a computer screen or on the phone. Residential care workers fill in endless forms. Everywhere, care work entails huge amounts of bureaucracy. New forms of management, audit, accountability, inspection and regulation have generated a vast edifice of technology which eats into precious time, leaving little spare to build relationships. In the last three decades, the bureaucracy has accumulated in response to every scandal and to the pressure to increase efficiency. The paperwork has become a way to avoid blame and manage risk. Sometimes, it is the main criteria by which care work is assessed and inspected, creating a cycle of behaviour which prioritizes bureaucracy over people. There is no shortage of rhetoric on the importance of the individual person, but despite all the good words and public pledges, the countervailing pressures to manage scarce resources compress opportunities for relationship, I was told again and again. These tendencies were already well entrenched by 2010, and the austerity which followed stripped staff resources to the minimum, making it all the more evident.

The marketization of care – in health and for the elderly – has led to a profound confusion around language, which is corrosive of meaning and purpose. Care is not a consumer product; it is always an encounter of one human being with another, and needs to be sustained by inspiration, ideals and example – in short, by the culture of the organization. John Kennedy, of the Joseph Rowntree Trust, urges organizations providing care to remember that they must always be vocational, their leadership explicit about the primacy of people.

Put blame, bureaucracy, marketization and technology together and the toxic combination stifles the authenticity, spontaneity and creativity essential to humanize care. No regulation or inspection can ever capture the value of this encounter described by a GP in the West Country: 'Last Friday afternoon I was doing a surgery which has a particular focus on mental health, self-harm and trauma; many of the patients who come are in contact with the criminal justice system. A woman was in complete physical and mental pain, an extreme case of Medically Unexplained Symptoms caused by multiple traumas in her life. There was nothing I could do. I couldn't even explain what I thought was going on; she was so emotionally distraught, she couldn't think straight. In the end, I sat down on another chair and turned my body round to face her and looked her in the eyes and just said, We are here with you. We will stay here. We won't reject you or say we can't help.

'It felt like the right thing to do. We don't understand the links between mind and body, and medicine runs out of answers, so all you have left is to demonstrate care. It's very painful, but I deal with it. I reset myself in that moment as someone who doesn't have answers, but makes some kind of commitment to not let her down, as she so often has been. She looked genuinely grateful.'

*

The crisis may get worse as the ageing population adds to the pressure on every part of the care economy, family and public. Other factors give cause for deep concern. Over the last two decades, debate on how to fund the care economy has been crippled by a reluctance to raise tax or establish mechanisms such as insurance to ensure higher contributions; Theresa May's attempt at a funding solution in the 2017 election has left the Conservative party wary of taking the bold action on social care that is required. In December 2019, care in one form or another was second only to Brexit as the most significant election issue; while the Conservatives promised 50,000 new nurses, Labour unveiled a raft of ambitious promises, including a National Care Service that would double the number of adults receiving free social care. The politics of care are likely to become more fraught as economic trends drive up the *relative* cost of care. The American economist William Baumol was the first to point this out in 1993: he argued that rising productivity would increase wealth threefold in the US as automation spread through manufacturing and agriculture, but he warned that productivity in health and education would grow more slowly – if at all – and remain labour-intensive, making these services relatively, and absolutely, more expensive. The means to pay for such services would be there, but it would be a matter of politics whether societies would agree to divert that wealth to cover the costs. According to Baumol's analysis, we are only in the foothills of an embittered politicization of care.

Another pressing cause for concern is that shortages in the care workforce, already a major challenge, will be exacerbated by the UK government's commitment to reduce migration. A striking characteristic of this country's care economy has been its historic dependence on migrant labour. From its inception, the NHS attracted nurses and auxiliaries from Ireland (in 1971 it was estimated that 12 per cent of nurses were Irish) and the

Caribbean, and in the 1960s 18,000 doctors were recruited from India and Pakistan. More recently, EU nationals have filled thousands of jobs. In 2012 over a fifth of the UK's nurses were born abroad, and over a third of doctors; in 2017 a House of Commons report said that 13.1 per cent of all NHS staff reported a non-British nationality. The comparable figures in France or Italy are much smaller; analysis points to a range of contributory factors such as a shortage of training places in the UK, an historic complacency that imported ready-trained staff to save on training costs, and a failure to make healthcare jobs sufficiently attractive. The situation is even more stark in social care; one fifth of all UK care workers were born abroad, with the largest numbers coming from India, Poland, the Philippines and Romania. This is particularly evident in London and the south-east, and more than half of all care workers in the capital are foreign-born.

There is a global shortage of health workers, and the UK faces growing competition from other countries such as Australia and the United States, which offer better pay and working conditions. Following the Brexit vote in 2016, a significant number of EU nationals have left, and new arrivals have dropped off. The UK government wants to put tight controls in place to further reduce migration and proposed in 2019 a salary threshold of £30,000 a year for skilled workers, effectively ruling out all care work and many junior healthcare positions. The route into the UK for low-skilled workers would be a twelve-month temporary visa, and agriculture would be the only exception. Such a proposal would choke off migrant recruitment, bringing care systems in places like London to crisis point, struggling to cope with high vacancies and reliant on an ever-changing pool of workers. The vacancy rate in care work is already 9 per cent, and such a tightening of immigration rules would be catastrophic.

At the point where recruitment should be rising in a range of health and care jobs, the supply of applicants is shrinking. When I began researching the subject of care in 2015, there seemed a chance of action, but the ongoing struggle over Britain's departure from the European Union has crippled any effective policy response. The issue has been stranded in a political no-man's land.

Hopes of an affordable health and care system increasingly focus on technology as the answer. Artificial intelligence and robotic technology are set to make dramatic breakthroughs in the next thirty years in many areas of life, and have the potential to offer a multitude of different applications. A breathless excitement characterizes the policy reports which promise that these developments will usher in a revolution in care. Across the world, robots are increasingly used in surgery, with fewer complications and greater safety; they are more dexterous and accurate in making knots and stitching. Artificial intelligence is being developed to improve diagnosis, and in some cases has proved to be more reliable; for example a new AI system, Lymph Node Assistant, can analyse slides and improve detection rates of breast cancer. Google DeepMind has started using AI to analyse CT and MRI scans from cancer patients to distinguish between healthy and cancerous tissue. These would be great breakthroughs, and many believe that aspects of healthcare such as pathology could become almost completely automated. Increasingly, algorithms will play a role in almost every area of diagnosis; a Danish software company applied a deep-learning programme to emergency calls. The algorithm analysed what the caller said, tone of voice, background noise, and detected cardiac arrests with a 93 per cent success rate, compared to 73 per cent for humans, and reached the decision faster.

'Telehealth' has great potential for the management of long-term conditions such as diabetes and heart disease; it entails combining digital platforms with sensors and implants to monitor treatment and gather data such as blood-sugar levels and heart rhythms. Some applications of telehealth have been developed for care of the elderly; one project with video software enables family members and care workers to provide medication reminders by video chat, while an integrated intelligent wristband detects falls and seizures, and monitors heart rate and skin temperature. Data-driven alerts come up on the caregiver's dashboard if anything appears to be wrong. The project suggests a possible future in which the care worker could be sitting in front of a bank of screens, monitoring dozens of elderly people in their own homes with real-time information on their health. The harassed relative could check in from their office desk to see that the elderly person has remembered medication or been drinking enough water.

Another frontier which is rapidly opening up is in the use of robots in home care. Already widespread in manufacturing, it is estimated that by 2040 robots will outnumber humans by 10 billion. They will be cleaning our homes, doing the washing up and perhaps bathing those stumbling into a frail old age. One company press release declared that robots will 'not just make eldercare viable and affordable in an otherwise bleak future', but 'give the elderly the level of attention and mobility they deserve and which humans can't really provide for them'. Care is being redefined as something humans are not good at, according to corporate PR which suggests robots are more attentive and more patient.

This future is not far away. Advances in the technology will ensure that robots can help with dressing, eating and toileting by 2021–5. Already a 'Care-o-bot' has been used in care homes in Germany to transport food and drinks and keep residents entertained with memory games. In the next fifteen years, robots will be able to provide 'safe, dexterous, close physical interaction for care and support', according to expert predictions. Breakthroughs are expected in how robotic systems map homes, recognize people and everyday objects, as well as in their capacity for dialogue and learning in the next few years. Before long, they will understand intentions and emotions, and plan complex tasks; within twenty years, it is predicted that robots will be capable of natural conversation and be able to give an account of their behaviour.

The country which has been at the forefront of how this technology could be applied to care is Japan. Ageing demographics in the country present a particular challenge because of a long-standing resistance to immigration to fill low-paid care jobs. Around £3.6 billion has already been invested, and robots are being used in hospitals and homes to lift patients and serve food. By 2020 four out of five care recipients in Japan will have some form of robotic support. One robot developed for the Japanese market is 'Robear', a robotic nurse capable of lifting a patient and washing their hair, while another, known as 'Pepper', is humanoid in appearance and has the power to read and respond to human emotions such as joy, surprise, anger, doubt and sadness. These robots are designed to be constantly learning and fine-tuning their responses to human emotion as interactions are uploaded to the cloud. One technological company claimed in its promotional material that 'robots are more patient than humans', and its chief executive assured prospective customers that his robots will be 'pure, nice and compassionate towards people'.

Huge enthusiasm greets the possibilities of this robotic technology and artificial intelligence; one influential report urged the NHS to adopt a 'tilt to tech' to reap 'an astonishing array of opportunities'. It went on to comment that 'tech has made consumer experience far faster, easier and more convenient. There is no reason that the NHS and social care can't make accessing services as easy as a few taps on an app.' It concluded, 'given the scale of productivity savings required in health and care – and the shortage of front-line staff – automation presents a significant opportunity to improve both the efficiency and the quality of care in the NHS'. Authored by a commission led by one of the most influential figures in UK health policy, Lord Ara Darzi – a surgeon who has pioneered the use of robotics – the report was designed to catch the eye of politicians, with a promise that automation would save the NHS £12.5 billion. It predicted 'smart homes that include point-of-care diagnostics together with remote monitoring, meaning that people will be able to live independently, secure in the knowledge that help is close at hand if their condition deteriorates. Robotics and virtual reality systems could be deployed to homes to deliver rehabilitation,' while Home Help Robots 'could help people to get out of bed, to wash and dress, to eat and drink, and with mobility and social engagement. Robots can help people maintain their homes … The future is full of possibilities where robots empower people in old age, enabling better, longer, and more fulfilling lives.' It went on to suggest that 'robots will enable people to remain more socially connected to friends and family'. It promised that 'automation will primarily complement human skills and talents, by reducing the burden of administrative tasks – communicating medical notes, booking appointments, processing prescriptions – while freeing up time for clinical decision making and caring.' The placing of this last word seemed cursory. The report barely referred to care beyond defining two attributes: access ('receiving the care required in a timely and convenient fashion') and quality, which it defined as 'safe and effective'. It called for 'care that is caring: providing services with compassion, dignity and respect', with little consideration as to how such characteristics would fit alongside the new technology. Care should entail 'an experience of interacting with services that is convenient and similar to the standards of service we would expect in other areas of life'. The sentence summarizes the contradictions care professions have to straddle, suggesting that, like Amazon Prime, a carer can be booked for next-day delivery. But compassion and convenience belong to two very different value systems. A commercialized consumer culture is deeply entrenched in our understandings of care, impoverishing and distorting the relationship, inflating expectations and generating resentment. This is not about either technology or relationship, but about recognizing the complexity of how the two interact, and according comparable levels of significance to both.

Another enthusiastic report advocating automation in the NHS promised that it would 'allow NHS staff more time to do the vital jobs they love' and that 'increased automation can also help to address staff shortages, as it frees healthcare professionals from more repetitive tasks and allows them to focus on patient care'. The report argued that the social-care sector could save £5.9 billion annually from accelerated automation, and cited Sir John Bell, Regius Professor of Medicine at Oxford University, who suggested that 'AI might be the thing that saves the NHS'. But it went on to acknowledge that 'empathy and compassion are key aspects of providing high quality services and highly valued by patients', and admitted that 'this will be a barrier to the wide-scale rolling out of automation'. It insisted this was 'not an insurmountable obstacle'; the tendency of humans to anthropomorphize robots and project human personalities on to them would facilitate their acceptance. Automation could lead to more human interaction, with robots performing tasks both carer and recipient found the most uncomfortable, such as toileting, thus freeing up time for conversation.

The blithe reassurances do not convince everyone. The leading UK research body into AI, the UK Robotics and Autonomous Systems Network (UK-RAS), acknowledges concern that technology could be used as a substitute for interaction with people, and suggests that there 'need to be safeguards to protect against threats such as a reduction in the human aspects of care'. Their report concludes that 'we consider it essential that there is always a human contribution in social care. Indeed we advocate legislation to protect the right to direct contact with human carers alongside the development of robotics and AI tech.' They warned that robotic and autonomous systems 'will not match or replace the ability of human carers in the near future. The interpersonal aspects of care such as empathy and understanding are uniquely human. AI personal assistants and social robots may be able to provide a form of synthetic companionship that people find engaging, but this will never replace human companionship.' Their sober words are a grim foretaste of some of the battles over care which may take shape in coming decades.

The American psychologist Sherry Turkle has been studying the impact of technology on people since the 1970s, and suggests that there has been 'a flight from conversation' in every area of our lives, as people turn to technology rather than dealing with the 'messy, and demanding' nature of face-to-face human inter-action. Technology – for example, dealing with email – gives a satisfying sense of being in control, all the more seductive in the context of providing care in a stressful situation. At the bedside, the patient's suffering and fear is palpable and one's ability to offer relief limited, but a few feet away at a desk in front of a computer, the uncomfortable emotions of helplessness can fade.

It has long been known that in contexts of high anxiety and stress – such as healthcare – institutions develop defence sys-tems to manage. In a groundbreaking study of nurses published in 1960, the psychoanalyst Isabel Menzies Lyth suggested a system of 'ritual task performance' had evolved, in which each nurse was taught to follow a rigid task list. Nurses were assigned a particular activity to be done for all patients – such as washing or feeding – thus reducing the time they spent with each individual patient and relieving them of the possibility of closer relationship. Other characteristics of nursing care included depersonalization – calling patients by terms such as 'liver in bed three', for example – as well as standardizing behaviour and routines to avoid decision-making, and reducing the burden of responsibility by checking and counterchecking. Menzies Lyth noted that a high proportion of nurses dropped out of training, feeling distanced from the caring relationship. Despite changes in the way nurses work, the continued relevance of Menzies Lyth's work is widely acknowledged; screen-based tasks may well serve as a welcome distraction from the deep anxiety she first identified in response to suffering, reinforcing their prevalence in the nurse's daily schedule. Adam Phillips and Barbara Taylor write about the 'disturbing tension that can be aroused when faced with extreme need', which can prompt a desire to escape. 'The urge to turn away can be overwhelming', because profound need confronts us with 'the fear that we are not equipped to meet it'. In such situations, replying to emails, inputting data and filling out forms can take precedence over a difficult conversation.

Turkle likens the impact of technology to a new 'silent spring', the term Rachel Carson coined about environmental damage, arguing that 'technology is implicated in an assault on empathy'. This is true of every age group, suggests Turkle; in studies of twelve-year-old school children, she found it 'a struggle to get the children to talk to each other in class, to directly address each other. They looked at their phones at lunch and when they share, they are sharing what's on their phones.' She comments that 'face to face conversation is the most human – and humanizing – thing we do. It is where we listen, develop the capacity for empathy and where we experience the joy of being heard and understood'; she warns that in the past twenty years, there has been a 40 per cent decline in the markers for empathy among college students, and most of that fall has been in the last ten years.

Another perspective on Turkle's 'silent spring' is provided by the work of the psychiatrist and scientist Iain McGilchrist. In his monumental study *The Master and His Emissary*, he drew on a lifetime of research and clinical practice to develop a set of ideas about how the human brain has two contrasting ways of thinking. Both are essential, but the development of Western culture has increasingly privileged one of these. They broadly correlate to the two hemispheres of the brain. The left brain tends to the abstract and instrumental, and produces confident, certain, task-oriented thinking, while the right brain is more contextual, tentative, intuitive and often inarticulate. These two develop distinctive patterns of attention – they notice different things. Western cultures have developed the left-brain way of thinking and can point to its significant achievements in science and technology, but the right brain is 'more accurate, more down to earth – in a word, truer', suggests McGilchrist. As the left brain dominates, it instrumentalizes, seeks to grasp ideas and things, it wants control and certainty. Whatever doesn't fit is 'simply declared meaningless'. The right brain produces those intuitive, imaginative responses found in the creative arts and mythology, which, he adds significantly, are essential to good care. It has the capacity to see the connections between seemingly disparate things, to imagine another person's experience and to see the bigger picture. 'One way of looking at the difference would be to say that while the left hemisphere's raison d'être is to narrow things down to a certainty, the right hemisphere's is to open them up to possibility.'

The left hemisphere uses things, seeing in everything a calculus of utility. It is good at manipulating them, but less good at explaining or understanding meanings. The left may be better with data – words and figures – but disregards the wisdom, often tacit, which is discovered by experience. It is the right hemisphere which sees how individuals are 'reciprocally bound in a network, based on a host of things that could never be rationalized'. With that comes an appreciation of being part of a 'living web of experience' rather than detached observers, a place of deep loneliness, he asserts. Importantly, one of McGilchrist's concerns is that the left-brain task orientation is strengthened by many forms of digital communication, which are designed to sustain concentration by providing quick psychological rewards, thus reinforcing this way of experiencing the world.

A famous psychological experiment illustrates aspects of his argument: two teams of students passed a ball back and forth, while the subjects of the experiment had to observe and record the movement of the ball. Halfway through the experiment, a student dressed in a gorilla suit ambled between the teams. Half of those surveyed were so intent on their prescribed task, they did not even notice the gorilla and, even more worrying, half of them refused to believe the gorilla had been there: we are not just blind, we are blind to our blindness. We can completely fail to see something that is right in front of us. As McGilchrist puts it: 'the nature of the attention we choose to pay alters the nature of the world we experience, and governs what it is we will find. This in turn governs the type of attention we deem it appropriate to pay. Before long we are locked into a certain vision of the world as we become more and more sure of what it is we see.'

The left hemisphere has proved a very powerful way of thinking, because it offers simple explanations and certainty, but to follow the implications of McGilchrist's argument, we risk losing the patterns of attention essential for many forms of care. He concludes that contemporary culture is 'the least perceptive, the most dangerous', because 'routes that used to lead out of the hall of mirrors have been cut off, undercut and ironized out of existence'.

Turkle imagines a dystopian future in which 'we expect more from technology and less from one another' and are drawn to technologies 'that provide the illusion of companionship without the demands of relationship'. In such a future, face-to-face contact with a carer could become a rare luxury for those who can afford it, while the rest have to make do with a digital platform, sensors and the synthetic companionship of AI.

What makes this a vivid possibility is that we have already started down this path. In recent decades the lack of relationship in the healthcare system has contributed to the growth of complementary medicine. With ten-minute GP appointments, those with enough money look elsewhere for attention and human interaction. There are estimated to be 150,000 therapists working in the UK, and that 16 per cent of the population have turned to acupuncture, massage, osteopathy and chiropractic treatments. This form of care is not cheap (often £70 per session) and can last for years. Typically appointments are for an hour, and the relationship with the practitioner is central and continuous. Those who can afford it will pay for relationships.

Scarcity of face-to-face care, loneliness and increasing reliance on technology is a plausible future, but it may not happen: an alternative is entirely possible. We could be on the cusp of a dramatic moment when the cultural value of care could be completely recast. While automation is predicted to make millions of jobs obsolete, most experts believe that care is one of the few areas of employment which will hold steady or even increase. As with plumbing, the job requires too much dexterity and complexity to make mass automation cost-effective. Andy Haldane, the chief economist to the Bank of England, estimates 15 million jobs lost, while the economist Adair Turner suggests that 'automation will be rapid, unstoppable and limitless', and that 'we are in the early stages of a technological revolution which will eventually result in the automation of almost all economic activity, almost all work activities. It is not if, but when.' Already, automation is transforming manufacturing and retail; a Shanghai fulfilment centre can now process 200,000 orders a day with just 4 employees, while Amazon has opened grocery stores without checkouts in San Francisco. The Adidas Speedfactory in Bavaria employs 160 workers to make 500,000 pairs of shoes a year. It has been estimated that self-driving cars will put 230,000 taxi drivers out of business in the UK. Jobs will disappear across manufacturing, warehouses, transport and retail. It is not just low-skilled work which will succumb to automation; white-collar professions such as law and accountancy are also highly vulnerable. Only a few areas will be resistant to full automation, the three Cs being uppermost: care, cooking and the creative industries. Most economists are sceptical about the excited predictions of automation in care, and argue that care work will become a rare area of *growing* employment. There has been a 20 per cent growth in the care workforce over the ten years 2009–19, and that is likely to continue.

Haldane points out that there will be a profound shift in the kind of skills required in this new economy. In the last 300 years, there has been a growing demand for cognitive skills – high and fast intelligence and good memory – and they have attracted better wages than technical skills or social skills. They have dominated educational systems, accumulating cultural prestige and authority. He characterizes this as the 'head' having dominated over the 'hands' and the 'heart'. That is about to change: 'In the century ahead, these skill-shifts may be about to go into reverse ... My reading of the runes is that there are three areas where humans are likely to preserve some comparative (if not always absolute) advantage over robots for the foreseeable future. The first is cognitive tasks requiring creativity and intuition ("heads"). These might be tasks or problems whose solutions require great logical leaps of imagination rather than step by step hill-climbing. The second area of prospective demand for human skills is bespoke design and manufacture ... The third, and perhaps the biggest potential growth area of all, is social skills ("hearts"). That is, tasks requiring emotional intelligence (such as sympathy and empathy, relationship-building and negotiation skills, resilience and character) rather than cognitive intelligence alone. These are skills a robot is likely to find it hard to replicate. And even if they could replicate them, humans might still prefer humans to carry them out. The future could see a world of work in which EQ rivals IQ for skill supremacy.'

Haldane predicts a rise in demand for jobs with high degrees of personal and social interaction, such as health, care, education and leisure. He suggests that jobs which have combined the cognitive and the social in the past might change so that the latter assumes more significance, and the cognitive part is automated. Picking the example of a doctor, he argues that their clinical competence may become less significant because diagnostic algorithms will be more effective, but patients will want the relationship with the doctor as much as ever. Haldane's thesis is echoed by others, including Adair Turner, who foresees expansion of just two types of jobs: the hi-tech and what he calls the 'hi-touch', which includes care and hospitality. The scientist Sir Martin Rees predicts that 'caring will be one of the great professions of the future'.

Most predictions of the impact of automation are accompanied by warnings of the social dislocation caused by large job losses and accelerating inequality. A small elite will have highly paid jobs generating economic wealth, to which large swathes of the population could have little access. The traditional model of work as a means of earning a living and achieving a sense of status and self-worth will be available only to a minority. Haldane fears that 'the societal costs of transition could be large, in terms of rising wage inequality, a falling labour share and damage to social cohesion'. Central tenets of orthodox economics will cease to be meaningful, argues Turner, such as GDP as a measure of progress or the preoccupation with productivity. 'Driving further productivity growth should no longer be a primary objective of policy,' Turner told an audience at Johns Hopkins University, Washington DC, in 2018; instead, 'we need to focus education around equipping people to lead fulfilled lives even when humanity's need to work has largely disappeared'. He urged a policy of adequate wages and status for caring services as 'jobs which deliver high inherent welfare benefits', and called for the necessary political decisions to ensure this could be funded. Mainstream economists such as Haldane and Turner are even considering proposals such as the Universal Basic Income – a flat-rate payment to everyone in a country – to maintain living standards when work no longer organizes our time. The principle of the work ethic to motivate people's efforts and distribute rewards is unravelling. In the reinvention of the meaning of a worthwhile life, care and creativity will be central. Ideas once on the margin are being taken up by mainstream economists.

Speaking on this subject at Oxford University in 2018, Haldane invited the higher-education sector to rethink its purpose. 'For decades, the primary focus of these institutions has been on providing young people with cognitive skills,' but in future as much emphasis or even more will need to be put on developing technical and social skills available throughout the life course: 'Head, hands and hearts sharing equal billing.' He challenged Oxford: what would it look like if emotional intelligence was at the heart of its degrees?

I glimpsed what such an education might look like in a college for social pedagogues in Denmark. In the early twentieth century, a movement across Germany, Poland and Scandinavia ambitiously reimagined care as a profession, and created the discipline of social pedagogy. The English dictionary defines 'pedagogy' as the method and practice of teaching, but in many European countries social pedagogy has a much wider meaning: the nurturing of human development at every stage of the life course. The central focus is on the development of relationships to allow the individual to flourish. Well-being and community development are interrelated, and human interaction with the world is through head, hands and heart. Social pedagogues work in a wide variety of contexts, ranging from childcare to community psychiatry and residential care homes for the elderly.

On a visit to Aarhus in Denmark, I visited a college where students were studying social pedagogy as a three-year degree; I wandered around halls and classrooms confused, wondering if I had inadvertently arrived in a creative-arts college. The walls were covered with paintings, several rooms were stacked with sculptures, ceramics, props and musical instruments. But no, this was how they trained social pedagogues, using dance, music, theatre and art as way to develop the students' sense of identity and their humanity. Later, they might take these creative skills into their work as pedagogues. Of these students, some would work with the elderly, some with children and others with people with disabilities or mental illness. All these disparate areas of care required the same set of skills – humanity, empathy, creativity – while the specialist knowledge could develop later.

I was taken on a tour to see how the social-pedagogy training influences the work. My first stop was to a children's care home, where the director, a pedagogue in his late fifties, sat me down at a table laid with coffee and cakes, and lit a candle (it was midwinter) and suggested we get to know each other. He went on to explain that if I wanted to understand his work, we needed to establish a relationship, and he asked me questions about myself. As teenage residents of the home and the staff wandered in and out of our meeting, he described his career and his understanding of social pedagogy. Training required a process of self-development, he suggested, in which one finds one's own gifts for nurturing other people. A social pedagogue needed creativity, autonomy, patience and, crucially, the ability to judge when to intervene and when to step back. All these skills were underpinned by daily or weekly meetings for reflection with colleagues to discuss cases. As we ate cake in the candlelight, I was impressed by this professionalization of care and the validation of the time and personal development required, but even he lamented that the tide of optimism of the 1960s and 1970s, with its vibrant faith in human nature, which had carried him into the profession, had receded.

My next visit was to a forest-school kindergarten outside Aarhus, where twenty children ranging from three to six years, dressed in padded winter suits, came every day to the woods – regardless of the weather. I was fascinated by the way the social pedagogues interacted with the children; they didn't set them tasks or activities, but allowed the children the space and freedom to create their own games, and only intervened subtly to pick up on and develop the children's ideas. Always, the emphasis was on collaboration – between social pedagogue and child, and amongst the children themselves. The result was a gentle, busy hum of children playing – with not a desk, ruler or whiteboard in sight. As the early Polish pedagogue Janusz Korczak put it, 'If you want to be a pedagogue you have to learn to talk with children instead of to them. You have to learn to trust their capabilities and possibilities.'

At the college, several of the social-pedagogy degree students had just completed a module of a social-work degree in the UK, and we talked about the contrasts between the two countries' training. They admitted they were puzzled by their

UK studies, which had been dominated by bureaucratic procedures and risk management. They had returned to Denmark with relief. What stayed with me from the Danish model of social pedagogy was how closely it linked care to creativity and personal development, grounding all three in curiosity and imagination. Social pedagogy recognizes the need for spontaneity and to accommodate the unpredictable; it advocates regular reflective discussion amongst staff to bring theory and practice together.

One can pick out projects in the UK which have pioneered ways to bring the focus of care back to relationships. 'Schwartz Rounds' have been used in thousands of hospitals as a way to help staff reflect on the emotional and social challenges of their work. They are named after Ken Schwartz, an American lawyer who left a legacy to foster compassion in healthcare; during his treatment for terminal lung cancer, he said he had discovered that what mattered most was not the surgical skill or new drugs but that his carers empathized in a way that gave hope and made him 'feel like a human being not just an illness'. The meetings are open to all medical staff and last an hour; three or four staff each describe an incident in their work and members of the audience then contribute comments from their own experience. It enables staff to reflect openly with colleagues, without the usual professional hierarchies and without having to solve problems. Deceptively simple, it helps to reduce stress and isolation, fosters collaboration and reminds staff of their best intentions. One of the main organizations which trains staff to conduct Schwartz Rounds is the Point of Care Foundation, dedicated to promoting and fighting for a better appreciation of care in the health system.

Another inspiring example, in the very different context of residential care, is Shared Lives Plus, where people with a spare room offer to host someone for a few nights or a few months or longer. Guests include people with disabilities, mental ill health or dementia, or an elderly person. The host can also offer care, for which they are paid. The scheme has helped build relationships, and all within the context of a home environment. It has spread across the country, with 10,000 Shared Lives carers hosting 14,000 people. Greater Manchester has set a target for 15 per cent of people with learning disabilities in the city to join the scheme.

Social prescribing is a scheme in use since the 1980s and is available in many GP surgeries. Given that around one in five of all patients in GP surgeries have primarily a social or emotional problem, healthcare staff can help patients get subsidized access to local community activities, such as cooking classes, gardening, choirs or sport. The Bromley by Bow Centre in London pioneered the approach, and staff work with patients over several sessions, putting them in touch with appropriate activities – anything from legal advice to swimming lessons.

Other countries have experimented with 'care currencies'. The ageing demographics of Japan, combined with the fact that many children don't live near enough to their parents to offer care, led to the development of *Fureai kippu*, 'Caring Relationship Tickets', which can be earnt by offering care to an elderly person nearby and then, in turn, your parents can 'buy' care near to them. In the US, Elderplan enables more able members to provide care to others in exchange for credits. Such a concept has been practised in Bali for centuries; alongside conventional cash, Bali has a system of *Narayan banjar*, which is understood as work for the community. A *banjar* consists of fifty to 100 families who decide together what work is required. Such schemes stimulate interactions 'experienced as qualitatively different from the real economy. They are powered by and reinforce a different motivation; they bring regard from the community. They are motivated by care for others and a sense of connection. They have reciprocity built into them,' comments the social scientist David Halpern.

Imagine how such initiatives could be multiplied and scaled up with the right kind of state support. The benefits flow in many directions – to the user first of all, but also to the community and to the tax payer, in costs saved down the line. An economic case can be made for investing in this kind of social infrastructure. The economist Jerome De Henau and the Women's Budget Group calculated that an investment of 2 per cent of GDP in the care economy would create 1.5 million jobs in the UK. The method usually adopted by governments to stimulate economic growth is investing in physical infrastructure but they claimed that investing in the care economy instead would create more jobs, with stronger knock-on effects on economic growth and debt reduction. They pointed out that the sector is more labour-intensive and distributes employment across all parts of the country rather than being concentrated in better-off areas. Such investment would have a larger impact on household income and would boost consumption. It would yield returns well into the future, with a society that was better educated, healthier and better cared for. Indeed, all the arguments made for protecting the defence industry as a major employer in economically deprived parts of the country are just as relevant to care. The study was a bold attempt to make the case, and parts of this thinking were reflected in the Labour Party's manifesto for the 2019 general election.

Radical economics is putting an entirely new – and welcome – focus on care as an essential human activity. One set of ideas has emerged around the 'foundational economy', the essential services on which day-to-day life depends, both material and social. It includes utilities such as water, gas and electricity, as well as education, health and care; together they are the 'infrastructure of everyday, the basis of well-being and should be citizens' rights'. Estimating that 40 per cent of the workforce across Europe is employed in the foundational economy, the network of academics argue that the role of the state should be reoriented to support and promote it. The ideas have been taken up by the Welsh government, attracted by the fact that the foundational economy is 'sheltered', in the sense that it is not subject to international competition. Unlike inward investment – for a car plant or steel works – production will not move to another country when offered cheaper labour or tax incentives. Investment in the foundational economy would also reach places which have historically lost out. The Welsh government is exploring how care could be done differently, and how you build capabilities and appreciation of care, paid and unpaid, as a vital contribution to local communities. The foundational economy is low risk, with a steady return on capital and a long time horizon. For these ideas to translate into policy, several shifts are seen as critical: local citizen participation to set the priorities; a system of licensing so companies making money in the foundational economy have to recycle some of their revenue back into the local area; and the encouragement of small and medium-sized private and social enterprises to ensure that more of the revenue generated is reinvested. Described as 'provincial radicalism', it proposes that 'we need to start from an argument that the care of vulnerable people matters and we can do it better'.

The history of the last 150 years has been marked by astonishing advances in care in Western European democracies. One of most significant achievements was the professionalization of nursing, which was essential to the transformation of hospitals from places of death and rampant alcoholism. In the UK another milestone was the founding of the welfare state by the post-war Labour government, with the state assuming responsibility for funding and organizing healthcare and social care. In the latter half of the twentieth century, there were huge developments in understanding disability, mental health and child development. The quality of care has been one of the most important measures of our sense of progress, essential to our self-respect and identity as a country; the opening of the 2012 Olympic Games, with its paean of praise to the NHS, was a reminder of how care is both an expression of solidarity and a powerful contributor to national identity.

What underpinned that provision of care as an entitlement of each citizen was a set of ideals grounded in two belief systems: Christianity and humanism. Both have served as powerful narratives to inspire and motivate care. Both argue for the inherent value of each individual life and for the actions necessary to support each person's flourishing and full development as part of a shared humanity. Both have been central to the politics of social democracy and its commitment to the post-war creation of the welfare state. As the old adage runs, the founding of the Labour Party owed as much to Methodism as it did to Marx.

But in *Homo Deus*, the historian Yuval Harari raises the frightening possibility that such systems of meaning may fragment without the pressing need for labour. As automation makes many millions redundant to the processes of wealth creation, how then will we value the worth of individual lives, he asks. Religions, he argues, are a form of ideology which 'sustain social order'. One of the essential aspects of any social order is how care is inspired and organized: who offers it and how those individuals are then supported so that they can continue to care. All faiths acknowledge that the work of care can come at the cost of the self: this was the ideal of service, in which the history of care work is rooted. With the decline in religious practice in the UK, what will define, promote and inspire the values of care? What will provide a bulwark against the values of consumerism and their mythology of materialism, success and the quest for personal identity? The values of the market, such as utility – how can I use this person, how do they provide benefit to me? – compromise personal relationships and bring a shift of emphasis from connectedness to individualism, from presence to image, and from the long view to the instant. Care is a casualty because it encumbers and compromises autonomy; it is stigmatized for its associations with dependence and suffering, old age and death.

Along the way, what is lost is the understanding of the power of care relationships, their capacity to forge some of the deepest and most meaningful connections. Care is a set of activities which, like music, poetry and art, makes us human: it reflects our capacity for tenderness and generosity, to reach beyond our own self-interest to serve the flourishing of another. The faith we are now in danger of losing is in ourselves. The risk is that we turn on ourselves the capitalist strategy of exploitation and extraction, offering our lives for public entertainment on social media. Capitalism is restless, constantly in search of new frontiers where it can establish monetary transactions from which profit can be extracted. In mature economies, one of the last frontiers is intimate relationship – both with ourselves and with others. There has been a slow abandonment of territory to a set of market values which are incompatible with care – a dismantling of barricades designed to defend the possibility of dependence, vulnerability, responsibility and generosity in human relationship.

We need to speak about care in a different language, instead of the relentless macho repetition of words such as 'efficiency', 'quality', 'driving', 'choice', 'delivery' and 'productivity'. In *The Gift*, the poet Lewis Hyde reflects on the dilemmas of the artist, and asks how artists are to explain their labour in a market economy which values their work so poorly. His conclusions are just as relevant to care, that close but poor relation of artistic creativity. A work of art exists simultaneously in two 'economies', he writes – a market economy and a gift economy; 'only one of these is essential, however: a work of art can survive without the market, but where there is no gift, there is no art'. Seeing care as a form of gift recognizes the autonomy and creativity of the carer. Hyde reminds us that we are given a gift. It cannot be bought or coerced. Hyde suggests that the art – or substitute here the word 'care' – that is important to us, 'which moves the heart or revives the soul or delights the senses or offers courage for living, that work is received by us as a gift received. Even if we have paid a fee at the door of the museum or concert hall, when we are touched by a work of art [or care] something comes to us which has nothing to do with price.'

Richard Titmuss's *The Gift Relationship* (published in 1970) drew on the example of voluntary blood donors to argue that 'a fundamental truth of human existence' was that 'to love oneself, one must love strangers', and that the good society was built on this insight. In contrast, 'the market was coercive, forcing people into situations that thwart their natural altruism' and denying people the 'right to give'. The GP Julian Tudor Hart argued that the NHS was a gift economy. This is widely recognized in many ways – hence the thank-you cards covering the walls of the hospital and the GPs' staffroom. Even the private care company acknowledges the role of generosity in care, as it reassures customers with the promise that its staff will 'go the extra mile'. Hyde argues that the 'mythology' of capitalism has established the getting of things rather than the giving of things as the mark of status, in contrast to the gift economies of many indigenous peoples. 'So long as these assumptions rule, a disquieting sense of triviality, of worthlessness, even, will nag the man or woman who labours in the service of a gift and whose products are not adequately described as commodities.' Art and care cannot be understood only in terms of the market and that 'places a constraint upon their merchandising'. Decent pay and conditions are vital for the carer, but so too is the cultural frame which recognizes care as a gift of relationship.

The gift economy of many indigenous societies shares three qualities, according to the theorist who first coined the term, Marcel Mauss: the obligation to give, the obligation to accept and the obligation to reciprocate. As Hyde says, the essential requirement of gift economies is that 'the gift must always move' and its spirit 'is kept alive by its constant donation'. That was exactly the understanding of Kelly, the care worker interviewed in Chapter 6, when she explained how she believed her commitment to good care might, in turn, ensure it was available to her in several decades' time. She did not mean a straightforward quid pro quo; rather she saw the gift economy working across generations and across society. Kelly was not alone, and many of the people I interviewed expressed similar sentiments. Every act of kindness or human warmth we receive is one we, in our turn, can give, so that care 'must keep moving'. The inspiration passes from one person to the next in a myriad of encounters – some are brief, some last a lifetime, few are forgettable. Yet this gift economy is buried, often silently held in people's hearts without any wider social affirmation, obscured by language, institutional structures, policy documents and a public debate dominated by scandal and blame. This gift economy, recognized and properly rewarded, is needed to reclaim care and to celebrate the imagination, courage and sheer hard work it entails. It can never be measured and is rarely adequately described – with the inspiring exceptions of artists such as Rego, Tolstoy and Roth – but it is the raw stuff of how we experience our own humanity and that of others.

Acknowledgements

Throughout the writing of this book, I've been inspired by friends. They generously offered thoughts and provided new insights, many agreed to be interviewed or shared their own dilemmas and struggles as carers. At other times, they sustained me during the arduous labours of book writing with company, solidarity, humour and warmth. I am grateful to all the members of the group of women with whom I crazily jump into the freezing waters of Hampstead Heath Women's Pond every Sunday morning; their camaraderie, bravery and energy are a constant – if occasionally intimidating – inspiration. That insane plunge into the murky depths represents an exhilarating moment of abandonment of complex family responsibilities, reducing all thought to one: It's cold! Thank you Gillian, Martina, Maggie, Polly, Mariana, Sally, Erin and Dom.

One person in particular has been a frequent source of encouragement, ideas and interest; Brigit has thought and lived so much of this book and many suggestions originated with her. In a friendship which began when our daughters were only a few months old, she has always been an inspiration. Thanks also to life-long friends – Kate, Lucy and Cathy – and to my sisters – Emily and Teresa. I'm very fortunate to have some remarkable aunts; they offer the perspective and wisdom of their years free of the expectations between parent and child. They have all helped me to think how care – giving and receiving – plays out over a lifetime; thank you in particular to Barbara and Annabel. I only hope I can offer something comparable to some of my fifteen nieces and nephews. The presence of my mother hovers over several chapters; I'm grateful for all her support and care.

Some men are every bit as engaged in this life's labour and I'm grateful in particular to Tom Salter and to Jock Encombe (including one conversation on a sunny Musselburgh beach); both have found themselves through life circumstances developing deep insight into this subject. My thanks also to James Marriott and Ramiro Ortega. I owe a huge debt to Jim, Chris and Sophie, Heather and Amina, without whom several chapters could not have been written. Finally, one of the inspirations behind this book is my husband Simon, a man who has dedicated his working life to care; in addition, his unquestioning commitment to sharing the care of our family has given me a freedom still rare for many women. I have also relied on the care of two men intermittently in the last few years, and have learnt much from both; my thanks to Chris Cullen and Xerxes Dalal.

Many others are owed thanks for their support and inspiration including: Henny Beaumont, Melissa Benn, Lisa Baraitser, Stephen Batchelor, Richard Byng, Rowena Chapman, Joanna Cook, Marion Coutts, Rachel Dedman, Sophie Duckworth, Odette Duerden, Charlotte Encombe, Mary Flatley, Jacqueline Gordon, Denis Pereira Gray, Alison Leary, Ian Noonan, Caroline Nicholson, Pauline Ong, Tim Owen Jones, Kristine Pommert, Fran Panetta, Brigid Philip, Columba Quigley, Anne-Marie Rafferty, Heather Richardson, Libby Sallnow, Gilly Thomas, Mayuri Vyas, Bernadette Wren. Thanks to Margot for her encouragement at a bleak point, reassuring me that this subject is so vast and so important that any of us attempting to name it end up feeling that our efforts fall short of our ambition.

My thanks to Paula Hyde and the University of Manchester for a research fellowship; Paula invited me to give a keynote speech at a conference early in the process of book writing which helped me develop the ideas. Thank you to Rana Mitter for chairing the live recording of a series of essays on care in 2016 for *BBC Radio Three* at the British Academy. The Kiln Theatre, Kilburn, London, took up the issue of care after my radio series and with Brent Council commissioned an exhibition curated by Rachel Dedman; it was a great pleasure to see how she brought her own interpretation of care – including activism and carnival – to the subject.

As ever, I owe a huge debt to my agent Sarah Chalfant, whose commitment to this book has been unwavering; her care has been invaluable at numerous points. The team at Granta are everything one could wish for in a publisher: Bella Lacey's editing is rigorous and dedicated, and her enthusiasm is unflagging. Copy-editor Daphne Tagg is exemplary.

Finally, my gratitude to my three children, Ellie, Luke and Matt, for all the richness of receiving and giving care that they have brought to the last twenty-five years, and to my husband Simon for his stalwart constancy, his steadiness of purpose and integrity. The book is dedicated to him.

Notes

All web addresses were last retrieved in December 2019.

Introduction

p. 2   '*The care of the elderly and long-term sick* ...' Carers UK, *Facts about Carers*, 2015, https://www.carersuk.org/for-professionals/policy/policy-library/facts-about-carers-2015; also, *State of Caring: A Snapshot of Unpaid Care in the UK*, 2019, http://www.carersuk.org/images/News__campaigns/CUK_State_of_Caring_2019_Report.pdf

p. 2   '*As lives lengthen, one in four women* ...' *Facts about Carers* 2015

p. 3   '*Women dominate caring professions* ...' Department of Education, *Ethnicity Facts and Figures*, 14 May 2019, https://www.ethnicity-facts-figures.service.gov.uk/workforce-and-business/workforce-diversity/school-teacher-workforce/latest

p. 3   '*The proportion of women in general practice* ...' Nick Bostock, 'The Rise of Women in General Practice', *GP*, 8 March 2018, https://www.gponline.com/rise-women-general-practice/article/1458988

1. The Invisible Heart

p. 11   '*One well-known cause* ...' Carers UK, *Valuing Carers*, 2015, https://www.carersuk.org/for-professionals/policy/policy-library/valuing-carers-2015

p. 11   *'it will double between 2016 and 2041 ...'* Office for National Statistics (ONS), *Living Longer: Caring in Later Working Life*, March 2019, https://www.ons.gov.uk/peoplepopulationandcommunity/ birthsdeathsandmarriages/ageing/articles/livinglongerhowour- populationischangingandwhyitmatters/2019-03-15#overview

p. 11   'The Lancet *projects that ...'* Cited in Joe Dromey and Dean Hochlaf, 'Fair Care: A Workforce Strategy for Social Care', *IPPR*, 25 October 2018, https://www.ippr.org/research/ publications/fair-care

p. 11   *'Historical surveys reveal ...'* Pat Thane and Lynn Botelho, *The Long History of Old Age* (Thames and Hudson, 2005)

p. 12   *'Care for the elderly ...'* See ONS, *Living Longer*, March 2019, https://www.ons.gov.uk/peoplepopulationandcommunity/ birthsdeathsandmarriages/ageing/articles/livinglongerhowour- populationischangingandwhyitmatters/2019-03-15; Carers UK, *State of Caring: A Snapshot of Unpaid Care in the UK*, 2019, http:// www.carersuk.org/images/News__campaigns/CUK_State_of_ Caring_2019_Report.pdf

p. 12   *'over a third of carers ...'* Carers UK, *Facts about Carers*, 2015, https://www.carersuk.org/for-professionals/policy/ policy-library/facts-about-carers-2015

p. 12   *'one in four women ...'* ONS, *Living Longer* March 2019

p. 12   *'the number of people with a long-term health condition ...'* Department of Health and Social Care, *Long Term Conditions Compendium of Information*, 30 May 2012, https:// www.gov.uk/government/publications/long-term-conditions- compendium-of-information-third-edition; also Diabetes UK, *Facts and Figures*, https://www.diabetes.org.uk/professionals/ position-statements-reports/statistics

p. 13   *'the consequence is that risks ...'* David Halpern, *The Hidden Wealth of Humans* (Polity Press, 2010)

p. 13   *'women's employment rates ...'* Barra Roantree and Kartik Vira, *The Rise and Rise of Women's Employment*, Institute of Fiscal Studies, 2017, https://www.ifs.org.uk/uploads/BN234.pdf

p. 14   *'Grandparents are an essential lifeline ...'* International Longevity Centre UK, *The Grandparent Army*, 21 February 2017, https://ilcuk.org.uk/the-grandparent-army/

p. 15   *'young adults live at home ...'* ONS, *Young Adults Living with Their Parents*, 15 November 2019, https://www.ons.gov.uk/peoplepopulationandcommunity/birthsdeathsandmarriages/families/datasets/youngadultslivingwiththeirparents

p. 16   *'domestic service was the largest ...'* Lucy Lethbridge, *Servants: A Downstairs View of Twentieth-century Britain* (Bloomsbury, 2013)

p. 17   *'care has been framed as instinctive ...'* Nancy Folbre, *The Invisible Heart: Economics and Family Values* (New Press, 2001)

p. 18   *' such generous offices we do them ...'* Mary Astell, *Reflections Upon Marriage* (1706)

p. 18   *'J. S. Mill wrote ...'* John Stuart Mill, *The Subjection of Women*, Longmans, Green, Reader and Dyer, 1869; http://library.umac.mo/ebooks/b32202945.pdf

p. 18   *'Home was to be ...'* Sharon Hays, *The Cultural Contradictions of Motherhood* (Yale University Press, 1998)

p. 19   *'Virginia Woolf subjected ...'* Virginia Woolf, 'Professions for Women', in *The Death of the Moth and Other Essays*, 1942; http://gutenberg.net.au/ebooks12/1203811h.html

p. 19–20 *'the feminist Wendy Whitfield ...'* Cited in Melissa Benn, *Madonna and Child: The Politics of Modern Motherhood* (Vintage, 1999)

p. 20   *'Despite the huge increase of women in paid work ...'* Anne McMunn, et al., 'Gender Divisions of Paid and Unpaid Work in Contemporary UK Couples', *Work, Employment and Society*, 2019, https://journals.sagepub.com/doi/abs/10.1177/0950017019862153?journalCode=wesa

p. 20   *'The difference is even more stark ...'* OECD, *Balancing Paid Work, Unpaid Work and Leisure*, 2018, https://www.oecd.org/gender/balancing-paid-work-unpaid-work-and-leisure.htm

p. 20   *'for limited purposes we may imagine ...'* Virginia Held, *The Ethics of Care: Personal, Political and Global* (Oxford University Press, 2005)

p. 21   *'Despite being the largest source ...'* Lethbridge, *Servants*

p. 21–2 *'far too little of its own servants ...'*, *'so entirely excluded from all familiarity ...'*, *'low, distant humming ...'* Ibid.

p. 22   *'Yet care work is the fastest-growing ...'* UK Commission for

Employment and Skills, *Working Futures, 2014–2024*, https://assets. publishing.service.gov.uk/government/uploads/system/uploads/ attachment_data/file/543301/WF_Headline_Presentation_v3.pdf

p. 22   '*In 2015 a team valued just the unpaid work ...*' Sue Yeandle and Lisa Buckner, University of Sheffield, *Valuing Carers*, Carers UK, 2015

p. 23   '*begun to think and define ourselves ...*' Michael Sandel, *What Money Can't Buy: The Moral Limits of Markets* (Farrar Straus Giroux, 2012)

p. 23   '*The Taylor model gives the false illusion ...*' Alison Leary, interview with author

p. 25   '*Blair's gambit was that only ...*' Will Davies, 'They Don't Even need Ideas', *London Review of Books*, 20 June 2019

p. 27   '*few tasks are more like the torture of Sisyphus ...*' Simone De Beauvoir, *The Second Sex* (Vintage, 2015)

p. 27   '*the problem lay buried ...*' Betty Friedan, *The Feminine Mystique* (Penguin, 2015)

p. 27   '*self-defeating trivialities ...*' Cited in Hilary Graham, 'Caring: A Labour of Love', in Janet Finch and Dulcie Groves (eds), *A Labour of Love: Women, Work and Caring* (Routledge & Kegan Paul, 1983)

p. 28   '*motherhood had been abandoned by feminists ...*' Maureen Freely, *What About Us? An Open Letter to the Mothers Feminism Forgot* (Bloomsbury, 1995)

p. 29   '*Childlessness has nearly doubled ...*' ONS, *Childbearing for Women Born in Different Years, England and Wales*, 2017, https://www.ons.gov.uk/peoplepopulationandcommu- nity/birthsdeathsandmarriages/conceptionandfertilityrates/ bulletins/childbearingforwomenbornindifferentyearsenglan- dandwales/2017

p. 29   '*There has been a marked shift ...*' Angela McRobbie, *Analysis*, BBC Radio 4, 13 December 2006

p. 30   '*At a conference on care ...*' Lisa Baraitser, et al., 'Who Cares? The Care Emergency and Feminist Responses', *Feminist Emergency*, International Conference, Birkbeck, University of London, audio available at https://backdoorbroadcasting. net/2017/06/feminist-emergency-international-conference/

p. 30   *'if women in their justifiable quest for equality ...'* Held, *Ethics of Care*

p. 31   *'Local authorities have suffered ...'* Dromey and Hochlaf, 'Fair Care'

p. 31   *'1.4 million elderly people ...'* Age UK, *Care in Crisis*, 2019 https:// www.ageuk.org.uk/our-impact/campaigning/care-in-crisis/

p. 31   *'Only one in seven local authorities ...'* UK Homecare Association, cited in Dromey and Hochlaf, 'Fair Care'

p. 31   *'estimated to affect up to 220,000 workers ...'* Communities and Local Government Committee, *Adult Social Care*, March 2017, https://publications.parliament.uk/pa/cm201617/cmselect/ cmcomloc/1103/110303.htm

p. 31   *'Enforcement of employment law ...'* 'Skills for Care', 2018, cited in Dromey and Hochlaf, 'Fair Care'

p. 32   *'9–13 per cent of care jobs ...'* Cited in ibid.

p. 32   *'nearly half of care workers leave ...'* Ibid.

p. 32   *'a study of suicide trends ...'* ONS and Public Health England, *Suicide by Occupation*, March 2017, https://www.ons.gov.uk/ peoplepopulationandcommunity/birthsdeathsandmarriages/ deaths/articles/suicidebyoccupation/england2011to2015

p. 32   *'vacancy rates ran at 7.8 per cent ...'* Skills for Care, *The State of the Adult Social Care Sector and Workforce in England*, October 2019, https://www.skillsforcare.org.uk/adult-social- care-workforce-data/Workforce-intelligence/publications/ The-state-of-the-adult-social-care-sector-and-workforce-in- England.aspx

p. 32   *'the average age has jumped to forty-seven ...'* NHS Digital, *Personal Social Services: Staff of Social Services Departments*, February 2018, https://digital.nhs. uk/data-and-information/publications/statistical/ personal-social-services-staff-of-social-services-departments

p. 32   *'An Ipsos Mori poll ...'* Ipsos Mori, 'Public Perceptions of the NHS and Social Care: General Election Polling 2019', December 2019, https://www.ipsos.com/ipsos-mori/en-uk/public- perceptions-nhs-and-social-care-general-election-polling-2019

p. 33   *'Nurses were also badly affected ...'* James Buchan and Ian Seccombe, *In Short Supply: Pay Policy and Nurse Numbers*,

Health Foundation, 2017, https://www.health.org.uk/publications/in-short-supply-pay-policy-and-nurse-numbers. A new pay deal agreed in 2018 for 6.5 per cent over three years will not reverse this deterioration, although it will help nurses' pay keep up with inflation.

p. 33   '*an 8 per cent fall in pay* ...' Full Fact, *Pay Rises: How Much Do Nurses, the Police, Teachers and MPs Get Paid?*, September 2018, https://fullfact.org/economy/pay-rises-how-much-do-nurses-police-teachers-and-mps-get-paid/

p. 33   '*With a sharp drop in applications* ...' House of Commons Health Committee, *Expand the Nursing Workforce*, 26 January 2018, https://www.parliament.uk/business/committees/committees-a-z/commons-select/health-committee/news-parliament-2017/nursing-workforce-report-published-17-19/

p. 33   '*The worst levels of pay* ...' Cited by the Early Years Alliance, *40 Per Cent of Childcare Workers on National Living Wage are Underpaid*, 2018, https://www.eyalliance.org.uk/news/2018/11/40-childcare-workers-national-living-wage-are-underpaid

p. 33   '*In 2017 a nursery manager's pay* ...' Ceeda, *The About Early Years Annual Report, 2017–18*, https://aboutearlyyears.co.uk/our-reports/

p. 33   '*as much as 81 per cent of the workforce* ...' Early Years Alliance, *Mental Health and the Early Years Workforce*, https://www.eyalliance.org.uk/mental-health-and-early-years-workforce

p. 33   '*The gap in funding the childcare system* ...' All Party Parliamentary Group on Childcare and Early Education, *Steps to Sustainability*, https://connectpa.co.uk/wp-content/uploads/2019/07/Steps-to-sustainability-report.pdf

p. 34   '*The problem with looking at childcare* ...' Sue Cowley, *Freeing the Angel*, https://suecowley.wordpress.com

p. 34   '*universal change in the way society* ...' Ceeda, *About Early Years*

(i) care

p. 38   '*Virgil saw care as so burdensome* ...' Warren T. Reich, *History of the Notion of Care*, Georgetown University, https://theology.georgetown.edu/research/historyofcare/classicarticle/

p. 39   '*Heidegger uses the word* Sorge ...' Winton Higgins, *A Path with Care*, unpublished paper; also, *The Dictionary of Untranslatables*, ed. Barbara Cassin (Princeton, 2014)

p. 40   '*the generational task of cultivating strength* ...' Erik Erikson, cited in Reich, *Notion of Care*

p. 40   '*everything that we do to maintain* ...' Joan Tronto, *Moral Boundaries: A Political Argument for an Ethic of Care* (Routledge, 1993)

p. 41   '*as much as care is labour* ...' Sara Ruddick, *Maternal Thinking: Towards a Politics of Peace* (Beacon Press, 1995)

p. 41   '*about doing something, making decisions* ...' Rollo May, cited in Reich, *Notion of Care*

p. 41   '*a relation in which the carer and the cared for* ...' Held, *Ethics of Care*

2. Maintenance Art

p. 44   '*creates the floor of everyone's self* ...' Wendy Hollway, *The Capacity to Care* (Routledge, 2006)

p. 44   '*she would know the care and love in her body* ...' Maurice Hamington, *Embodied Care* (University of Illinois Press, 2004)

p. 45   '*know certain things about their surroundings* ...' Iris Murdoch, *The Sovereignty of the Good*, (Routledge & Kegan Paul, 1970)

p. 45   '*Care is a politically embodied performance* ...' Maurice Hamington, 'A Father's Touch: Caring Embodiment and A Moral Revolution', in Greg Johnson, et al. (eds), *Revealing Male Bodies* (Indiana University Press, 2002)

p. 46   '*being there to be left* ...' Erna Fullman, quoted in Lisa Baraitser, *Maternal Encounter: The Ethics of Interruption* (Routledge, 2008)

p. 47   '*somehow culturally buried* ...' Melissa Benn, *What Should We Tell Our Daughters? The Pleasures and Pressures of Growing up Female* (Hodder & Stoughton, 2013)

p. 47   '*were schooled in toughness* ...' Melissa Benn, *Madonna and Child: Towards a New Politics of Motherhood* (Jonathan Cape, 1998)

p. 48   '*it was a relief when they went to bed* ...' Virginia Woolf, *To the Lighthouse* (Hogarth Press, 1927)

p. 49   '*A willingness to be interrupted* ...' Baraitser, *Maternal Encounters*

p. 49　　*'shadow of clock time ...'* Valerie Bryson, *Gender and the Politics of Time* (Policy Press, 2007)

p. 50　　*'The rhythms of women's work ...'* E. P. Thompson, *'Time, Work-Discipline and Industrial Capitalism'*, Past & Present, 38:1, December 1967

p. 50　　*'one of the most basic social conventions ...'* Johan Goudsblom, cited in Bryson, *Gender*

p. 50　　*'Speed increasingly carries cultural prestige ...'* John Tomlinson, *The Culture of Speed: The Coming of Immediacy* (Sage, 2007)

p. 51　　*'battle between two kinds of time ...'* Bob Dylan, *Chronicles: Volume One*, cited in Bryson, *Gender*

p. 51　　*'attention to small chores, errands ...'* Adrienne Rich, *On Lies, Secrets and Silence* (W. W. Norton & Co., 1979)

p. 52　　*'Proposal for an Exhibition entitled Care ...'* Mierle Laderman Ukeles, *Maintenance Art Manifesto 1969*, http://www.queensmuseum.org/wp-content/uploads/2016/04/Ukeles_MANIFESTO.pdf; also https://www.tabletmag.com/jewish-arts-and-culture/138254/mierle-laderman-ukeles

p. 56　　*'who shall do what for whom ...'* Arthur Kleinman, *Illness Narratives: Suffering, Healing and the Human Condition* (Basic Books, 1988)

p. 57　　*'is held up in its buoyancy ...'* Iain Crichton Smith, *Towards the Human* (Saltire Society, 1988)

p. 57　　*'Marion Coutts captures this sentiment ...'* Marion Coutts, *The Iceberg: A Memoir* (Atlantic, 2014)

p. 57　　*'the most delicate and evanescent of moments ...'* James Joyce, *Stephen Hero* (Jonathan Cape, 1944)

p. 58　　*'There is no more sombre enemy of good art ...'* Cyril Connolly, *The Enemies of Promise: Charlock's Shade* (Routledge, 1938)

p. 58　　*'literature does its best to maintain ...'* Virginia Woolf, *On Being Ill* (Hogarth Press, 1930)

p. 60　　*'our remote obfuscating language ...'* Norman Doidge, 'How Oliver Sacks Put a Human Face on the Science of the Mind', *The Globe and Mail*, 5 February 2016, https://www.theglobeandmail.com/arts/books-and-media/awakenings-how-oliver-sacks-put-a-human-face-on-the-science-of-the-mind/article28599283/

p. 60   '*I am not her carer...*' Alan Bennett, *The Lady in the Van* (Profile Books, 1999)

p. 60   '*ideas become unimaginable...*' George Orwell, *Nineteen Eighty-Four* (Secker and Warburg,1949; Penguin, 2004)

p. 61   '*We need words to keep us human...*' Michael Ignatieff, *The Needs of Strangers* (Viking, 1985)

p. 61   '*I'm listening with my eyes and ears...*' Participant at *Performing Care* symposium, Royal Central School of Speech and Drama, 15 December 2016

p. 62   '*For his excretions also special arrangements had to be made...*' Leo Tolstoy, *The Death of Ivan Ilyich* (1886); available on https://www.ccel.org/ccel/tolstoy/ivan.txt

(ii) empathy

p. 66   '*moral test of our times...*' Barack Obama, speech at K.I.D.S/Fashion Delivers, 2006, https://www.youtube.com/watch?v=4md_A059JRc

p. 66   '*Empathy requires us to do something...*' Brene Brown on Empathy, *RSA Shorts*, 2013, https://www.youtube.com/watch?v=1Evwgu369Jw

p. 66   '*The word "empathy" was only coined...*' Susan Lanzoni, 'A Short History of Empathy', *The Atlantic*, 15 October 2015, https://www.theatlantic.com/health/archive/2015/10/a-short-history-of-empathy/409912/

p. 67   '*ability to appreciate the other person's feelings...*' Ibid.

p. 67   '*The word's meaning has shifted...*' Cited in Rae Grainer, '1909: The Introduction of the Word "Empathy" into English', *BRANCH: Britain, Representation and Nineteenth-Century History*, ed. Dino Franco Felluga (extension of *Romanticism and Victorianism on the Net*), http://www.branchcollective.org/?ps_articles=rae-greiner-1909-the-introduction-of-the-word-empathy-into-english

p. 67   '*it entailed four characteristics...*' Theresa Wiseman, *Journal of Advanced Nursing*, 23: 6 June 1996

p. 68   '*One NHS policy instructed nurses...*' John Carvel, 'Nurses to be Rated on How Compassionate and Smiley They Are', *Guardian*, 18 June 2008, https://www.theguardian.com/society/2008/jun/18/nhs60.nhs1

p. 68   *'Perhaps these expectations of demonstrating emotion ...'* J. Ward, et al., 'The Empathy Enigma', *Journal of Professional Nursing*, 28:1, Jan–Feb 2012, https://www.ncbi.nlm.nih.gov/pubmed/22261603

p. 68   *'I take care of people I can't stand ...'* Cited in Siobhan Nelson and Suzanne Gordon (eds), *The Complexities of Care: Nursing Reconsidered* (Cornell, 2000)

p. 68   *'if physicians are to be effective ...'* Gavin Francis, 'Why Physicians need "right compassion"', *New York Times*, 26/27 December 2015

p. 68   *'are taught how to* perform *the role ...'* Raymond Tallis, *Hippocratic Oaths: Medicine and Its Discontents* (Atlantic, 2004)

p. 69   *'The minds of men are mirrors to one another ...'* *Stanford Encyclopedia of Philosophy*, https://plato.stanford.edu/entries/emotions-17th18th/LD8Hume.html#SymCom

p. 69   *'we can do without it ...'* Woolf, *On Being Ill*

p. 70   *'Martha Nussbaum takes a different stance ...'* Martha Nussbaum, *Political Emotions: Why Love Matters for Justice* (Belknap Press, 2013)

3. Listening to Vivaldi

p. 73   *'at the same time I have to see the child ...'* Eve Feder Kittay, *Love's Labor: Essays on Women, Equality and Dependency* (Routledge, 1999)

p. 81   *'a savagely critical report ...'* Parliamentary Joint Committee on Human Rights, *The Detention of Young People with Learning Disabilities and/or Autism*, November 2019, https://www.parliament.uk/business/committees/committees-a-z/joint-select/human-rights-committee/news-parliament-2017/detention-learning-disabilities-autism-young-people-report-published-19-20/

p. 83   *'The number of nurses trained in learning disabilities ...'* Rebecca Gilroy, 'Learning Disability Care Facing a "Crisis" Following 40% Drop in Nurses', *Independent Nurse*, 15 August 2018, http://www.independentnurse.co.uk/news/learning-disability-care-facing-a-crisis-following-40-drop-in-nurses/180928/

p. 83   *'a survey of social workers . . .'* Care and Support Alliance, *Social Workers Speak Out*, 2017, http://careandsupportalliance.com/social-workers-speak-out-report-from-the-care-and-support-alliance/

p. 83   *'picked up at the earliest point . . .'* National Autistic Society, *Autism: Overview of UK Policy and Services*, 2016, https://dera.ioe.ac.uk/26154/2/CBP-7172_Redacted.pdf

p. 83   *'The average wait for a diagnosis of autism . . .'* National Autistic Society, *School Report 2016*, https://www.autism.org.uk/get-involved/media-centre/news/2016-09-02-school-report-2016.aspx

p. 84   *'By late 2018, it was reported that councils . . .'* Chaminda Jayanetti and Michael Savage, '"Devastating" Cuts Hit Special Educational Needs', *Observer*, 10 November 2018, https://www.theguardian.com/education/2018/nov/10/councils-face-crisis-special-needs-education-funding

p. 85   *'Gatekeeping, managing the queue . . .'* Hilary Cottam, *Radical Help*, Virago, 2018

p. 85   *'Cuts left social workers with large caseloads . . .'* Luke Haynes, 'Majority of Social Workers Looking to Leave Their Job Within the Next 16 Months', *Community Care*, 30 October 2018, https://www.communitycare.co.uk/2018/10/30/majority-social-workers-looking-leave-job-within-next-16-months-says-new-research/

p. 85   *'40 per cent of social workers . . .'* Ibid.

p. 85   *'the turnover rate . . .'* Charlotte Carter, 'Adult Care Staff Turnover Rises for Sixth Consecutive Year', *Community Care*, 4 October 2019, https://www.communitycare.co.uk/2019/10/04/adult-care-staff-turnover-rises-sixth-consecutive-year-report-finds/

p. 86   *'State services are apt to be blunt . . .'* Sydney Webb, cited in Cottam, *Radical Help*

p. 87   *'twentieth-century bureaucracies . . .'* Hannah Arendt, *On Violence* (Harcourt, Brace, Jovanovich, 1970)

p. 87   *'technical expertise gets prioritized . . .'* David Runciman, *How Democracy Ends* (Profile, 2018)

p. 88   *'75 per cent of the British workforce . . .'* Penelope Ismay,

Trust Among Strangers: Friendly Societies in Modern Britain (Cambridge University Press, 2018)

(iii) kindness

p. 96   '*frequent sense that kindness is the junior partner ...*' John Ballat and Penelope Campling, *Intelligent Kindness: Reforming the Culture of Healthcare* (RCPsych Publications, 2011)

p. 97   '*people are leading secretly kind lives ...*' Adam Phillips and Barbara Taylor, *On Kindness* (Hamish Hamilton, 2009)

p. 98   '*We need institutions and cultures ...*' Jonathan Tomlinson, 'Do Doctors Need to be Kind?', *A Better NHS*, 4 May 2012, https://abetternhs.net/2012/05/04/kindness/

4. Care as Dark Matter

p. 100   '*Nurses (predominantly women) are the backbone ...*', Full Fact, *The Number of Nurses and Midwives in the UK*, 23 January 2018, https://fullfact.org/health/number-nurses-midwives-uk/

p. 100   '*Demand on the NHS is rising sharply ...*' NHS Confederation, *NHS Statistics, Facts and Figures*, 14 July 20017, https://www.nhsconfed.org/resources/key-statistics-on-the-nhs

p. 100   '*More nurses are leaving the profession ...*' Jake Beech, et al., *Closing the Gap*, Health Foundation, King's Fund and Nuffield Trust, March 2019, https://www.health.org.uk/publications/reports/closing-the-gap

p. 100   '*Between 2009 and 2016 ...*' The number dropped from 604 to 576. See Richard Murray, *Falling Number of Nurses in the NHS Paints a Worrying Picture*, King's Fund, 12 October 2017, https://www.kingsfund.org.uk/blog/2017/10/falling-number-nurses-nhs-paints-worrying-picture

p. 101   '*now almost half that in Sweden ...*' Eurostat, *Healthcare Personnel Statistics*, November 2019, https://ec.europa.eu/eurostat/statistics-explained/index.php/Healthcare_personnel_statistics_-_nursing_and_caring_professionals

p. 101   '*learning disability (which fell by 41 per cent) ...*' Mimi Launder, '"Urgent Investment" Needed in Learning Disability Nursing', *Nursing in Practice*, 21 June 2019, https://www.

nursinginpractice.com/urgent-investment-needed-learning-disability-nursing-warns-rcn

p. 101   '*mental health (which fell by 10.6 per cent) ...*' Mental Health Network, 'Drop in Mental Health Nurses Shows NHS under "Severe Strain"', NHS Confederation, 27 September 2018, https://www.nhsconfed.org/news/2018/09/drop-in-mental-health-nurses-shows-nhs-under-severe-strain

p. 101   '*the nursing workforce is ageing ...*' Royal College of Nursing, *The UK Nursing Labour Market Review 2017*, https://www.rcn.org.uk/professional-development/publications/pub-006625

p. 101   '*nursing workforce needs to be expanded ...*' House of Commons Health Committee, *Expand the Nursing Workforce*, 26 January 2018, https://www.parliament.uk/business/committees/committees-a-z/commons-select/health-committee/news-parliament-2017/nursing-workforce-report-published-17-19/

p. 101   '*The scandal of the ...*' Report of the Mid Staffordshire NHS Foundation Trust Public Inquiry, 6 February 2013, https://www.gov.uk/government/publications/report-of-the-mid-staffordshire-nhs-foundation-trust-public-inquiry

p. 101   '*But as one report concluded ...*' Jenny Firth-Cozens and Jocelyn Cornwall, *Point of Care*, King's Fund, 2009

p. 102   '*a series of moving articles on care ...*' Christina Patterson, *Healthcare: Nursing and the NHS*, https://christinapatterson.co.uk/healthcare/

p. 102   '*socially valued place and distinctive identity ...*' Siobhan Nelson and Suzanne Gordon (eds), *The Complexities of Care: Nursing Reconsidered* (Cornell, 2006)

p. 102   '*Nursing has been idealized ...*' Gosia Brykczynska (ed.), *Caring: The Compassion and Wisdom of Nursing* (CRC Press, 1996), and Suzanne Gordon, *Nursing Against the Odds* (Cornell, 2006)

p. 102   '*must make no demand upon the patient ...*' Florence Nightingale, *Notes on Nursing: What It Is and What It Is Not*, 1859

p. 103   '*particularly blind to the contribution ...*' Ann Oakley, *Taking it Like a Woman* (Jonathan Cape, 1984)

p. 103   '*leave nurses and nursing with no line of defence ...*' Nelson and Gordon, *Complexities of Care*?

p. 110   '*The number of hospital beds ...*' Nuffield Trust, *Hospital Bed*

Occupancy, 26 April 2019, https://www.nuffieldtrust.org.uk/resource/hospital-bed-occupancy

p. 111   *'only 40 per cent of a nurse's time ...'* Prime Minister's Commission, *The Future of Nursing and Midwifery*, 2010, https://webarchive.nationalarchives.gov.uk/20100331110440/http://cnm.independent.gov.uk/the-report/

p. 111   *'the common denominator ...'* Ibid.

p. 111   *'the word "basic" is used in a meaningless way ...'* Debbie Field, cited in Lisa Baraitser, et al., 'Who Cares? The Care Emergency and Feminist Responses', *Feminist Emergency*, International Conference, Birkbeck, University of London, audio available at https://backdoorbroadcasting.net/2017/06/feminist-emergency-international-conference/

p. 111   *'The loudest message we heard ...'* Prime Minister's Commission, *The Future of Nursing*

p. 111   *'as nursing becomes more academic ...'* Firth-Cozens and Cornwell, *Point of Care*

p. 112   *'we simply do not know whether the public ...'* Prime Minister's Commission, *The Future of Nursing*

p. 113   *'commodified view of need ...'* Penelope Campling, 'Reforming the Culture of Healthcare: The Case for Intelligent Kindness', *BJPsych Bulletin*, February 2015, https://www.cambridge.org/core/journals/bjpsych-bulletin/article/reforming-the-culture-of-healthcare-the-case-for-intelligent-kindness/61BE20409A5D80340AC35BFD437A23A2

p. 113   *'Not everything can be counted ...'* Nelson and Gordon, *Complexities of Care*

p. 113   *'Best known of all Florence Nightingale's books ...'* Mark Bostridge, *Florence Nightingale* (Viking, 2008)

p. 117   *'work of genius ...'* Cited in ibid.

p. 118   *'To many of the wounded and sick, especially ...'* Walt Whitman, *Memoranda During the War 1875–6*, https://whitmanarchive.org/published/other/memoranda.html.

p. 118   *'as carefully as a general ...'* Roy Morris Jr., *The Better Angel: Walt Whitman in the Civil War* (Oxford University Press, 2000)

p. 118   *'to give identity to the lives ...'* Walt Whitman, *Memoranda*

p. 119   *'Most of the actual nursing in the Crimea ...'* Anne Marie Rafferty, et al., *An Introduction to the Social History of Nursing* (Routledge, 1988)

p. 120   '*occurred wholly within a framework* ...' Siohban Nelson, *Say Little, Do Much: Nursing, Nuns and Hospitals in the Nineteenth Century* (University of Pennsylvania Press, 2001)

p. 120   '*nurses came to be known as "sisters"* ...' Rafferty, et al., *Social History of Nursing*

p. 120   '*the family circle which her taste and talents* ...' Cited in Bostridge, *Florence Nightingale*

p. 121   '*by the end of the nineteenth century* ...' John Pierson, *Understanding Social Work: History and Context* (Open University Press, 2011)

p. 121   '*all the softness and gentleness of her sex* ...' Peter Benson Maxwell, cited in Bostridge, *Florence Nightingale*

p. 121   '*saint, completely led by God* ...' Elizabeth Gaskell, cited in ibid.

p. 125   '*Professionalization of caring* ...' Gosia Brykczynska (ed.), *Caring: The Compassion and Wisdom of Nursing* (CRC Press, 1996)

p. 125   '*One nursing academic described* ...' *Performing Care* symposium, Royal Central School of Speech and Drama, 15 December 2016

p. 125   '*In another example, a patient had spilled* ...' Sanchia Aranda and Rosie Brown, 'Ethical Expertise and the Problem of the Good Nurse', in Nelson and Gordon, *Complexities of Care*

p. 126   '*Nurses are still the profession most trusted* ...' Ipsos Mori, *Veracity Index*, November 2019

p. 127   '*Valerie Isles makes a distinction* ...' Valerie Isles, 'The Simple Hard and the Complicated Easy', *Really Learning*, http://www.really-learning.com/the-simple-hard-and-the-complicated-easy/

p. 127   '*when efficiency is pursued through the gathering* ...' Suzanne Gordon, https://suzannecgordon.com; and Gordon, *Nursing Against the Odds*

p. 133   '*The first revelation was the astonishing power* ...' George Monbiot, 'Through My Cancer, I Have Found the Key to a Good Life', *Guardian*, 8 May 2019, https://www.theguardian.com/commentisfree/2018/may/08/my-prostate-cancer-surgery-key-to-good-life

(iv) compassion

p. 134   '*We ensure that compassion is central . . .*' Department of Health, *Hard Truths: The Journey to Putting Patients First*, January 2014, https://assets.publishing.service.gov.uk/government/ uploads/system/uploads/attachment_data/file/270368/34658_ Cm_8777_Vol_1_accessible.pdf

p. 135   '*In the Tibetan Buddhist tradition . . .*' Interview with Buddhist teachers Akincano and Stephen Batchelor

p. 135   '*Compassion can easily be marginalized . . .*' Paquita de Zuleta, 'Compassion in Healthcare', *Clinical Ethics*, November 2013, https://journals.sagepub.com/doi/ full/10.1177/1477750913506484

5. Three Hundred Decisions a Day

p. 137   '*Every working day, nearly a million patients . . .*' NHS England, *NHS Survey says nine out of ten patients have 'confidence and trust' in their GP*, 11 July 2019, https://www.england.nhs.uk/2019/07/ nine-out-of-10-patients-have-confidence-and-trust-in-their- gp/

p. 137   '*Of those million daily appointments . . .*' Raymond Tallis, *Hippocratic Oaths: Medicine and Its Discontents* (Atlantic, 2004)

p. 138   '*demand is rising . . .*' British Medical Association, *General Practice in the UK: Background Briefing*, April 2017, pdf from www.bma.org.uk

p. 138   '*The shortfall is predicted to triple . . .*' 'GP Shortages: A Symptom That Won't Go Away', *Guardian*, 9 May 2019, https://www. theguardian.com/commentisfree/2019/may/09/the-guardian- view-on-gp-shortages-a-symptom-that-wont-go-away; and Billy Palmer, *Is the Number of GPs Falling Across the UK?*, Nuffield Trust, 8 May 2019, https://www.nuffieldtrust.org.uk/ news-item/is-the-number-of-gps-falling-across-the-uk

p. 138   '*Without GPs to staff them . . .*' Lea Legraien, 'Revealed: More Surgeries Than Ever Closed Last Year,' *Pulse*, 31 May 2019, http://www.pulsetoday.co.uk/hot-topics/stop-practice-closures/ revealed-more-surgeries-than-ever-closed-last-year/20038773. article

p. 138–9   '*one in five GPs do more than fifty consultations ...*' Julia Gregory, 'GPs Have Almost Twice the Safe Number of Patient Contacts a Day, *Pulse*, 18 January 2018, http://www.pulsetoday.co.uk/home/finance-and-practice-life-news/gps-have-almost-twice-the-safe-number-of-patient-contacts-a-day/20035863.article

p. 139   '*Following the horrific crimes ...*' Part of what made the Shipman case so disturbing was that many of his patients believed him to be a very caring and attentive doctor; he masked his actions beneath an avuncular, kindly manner.

p. 140   '*They suggested I sat in on consultations ...*' My presence was explained and patients were given the option to ask me to leave the room.

p. 142   '*fathomless aquifers of implicit knowledge ...*' Tallis, *Hippocratic Oaths*

p. 142   '*85 per cent of the evidence ...*' Ibid.

p. 143   '*even in this highly technical age ...*' Jonathan Tomlinson, *A Better NHS*, https://abetternhs.net/about/

p. 143   '*it lags well behind consultation times ...*' Greg Irving, et al., 'International Variations in Primary Care Physician Consultation Time', *BMJ Open*, 7:10, https://bmjopen.bmj.com/content/7/10/e017902

p. 143   '*according to an NHS survey ...*' Ruth Robertson, et al., *Public Satisfaction with the NHS and Social Care in 2018*, King's Fund, 2019, https://www.kingsfund.org.uk/publications/public-satisfaction-nhs-social-care-2018

p. 144   '*An extraordinarily high and sustained rate ...*' Julian Tudor Hart, *The Political Economy of Health Care* (Policy Press, 2010)

p. 145   '*where the vast, undifferentiated mass of human distress ...*' Iona Heath, *The Mystery of General Practice*, Nuffield Trust, 1995, https://www.nuffieldtrust.org.uk/research/the-mystery-of-general-practice

p. 145   '*all truths about disease ...*' E. J. Cassell, *The Nature of Suffering and the Goals of Medicine* (Oxford University Press, 2004)

p. 145   '*never achieve the virtual certainty ...*' Tudor Hart, *Political Economy of Health Care*

p. 151   '*What is the effect of facing ...*' John Berger, *A Fortunate Man: The Story of a Country Doctor* (Canongate, 2015)

p. 156   '*the luxury of being useful* ...' Cited in Gaby Hinsliff, 'Why Shouldn't the Over-50s Start a New Career?' *Guardian*, 25 November 2016, https://www.theguardian.com/commentisfree/2016/nov/25/over-50s-new-career-teacher

p. 160   '*doctors come a close second to nurses* ...' Ipsos Mori, *Veracity Index*, November 2019

p. 162   '*Medicine is changing from a craft* ...' Steve Iliffe, *From General Practice to Primary Care: The Industrialization of Family Medicine* (Oxford University Press, 2008)

p. 163   '*Commercializing and industrializing processes* ...' Tudor Hart, *Political Economy of Healthcare*

p. 163   '*lagged behind other service industries* ...' King's Fund, *Improving the Quality of Care in General Practice*, 2011

p. 164   '*Only recently has a study managed to demonstrate* ...' Isaac Barker, et al., 'Association Between Continuity of Care in General Practice and Hospital Admissions', *BMJ*, February 2017

p. 164   '*logic of choice* ...' Annemarie Mol, *The Logic of Care: Health and the Problem of Patient Choice* (Routledge, 2008)

p. 166   '*being a businessman, missionary or socialist* ...' Dr Margaret McCartney, 'Farewell Doctor Finlay', *BBC Radio 4*, January 2017, https://www.bbc.co.uk/programmes/b07j7nty

(v) pity

p. 168   'Pitie *was the word used by* ...' *Internet Encyclopedia of Philosophy*, https://www.iep.utm.edu/rousseau/

p. 169   '*it was a distinction and a mournful pleasure* ...' Gwen Raverat Darwin, *Period Piece: A Cambridge Childhood* (Faber, 1952)

6. Bearing Witness

p. 180   '*It works out at only £8.50 an hour* ...' All figures were given in 2017, before the latest implementation of the National Living Wage.

p. 181   '*more than half of social-care providers* ...' Hft, *Sector Pulse Check*, cited in Liam Kay, 'More Than Half of Social Care Providers "Handing Contracts Back to Local Authorities"', *Third Sector*, 12 February 2019, https://www.thirdsector.co.uk/half-social-

care-providers-handing-contracts-back-local-authorities/finance/
article/1525528

p. 181 *'The brunt of cuts in social-care budgets ...'* Richard
Humphries, et al., *Social Care for Older People: Home
Truths*, King's Fund and Nuffield Trust joint report, 15
September 2016, https://www.nuffieldtrust.org.uk/research/
social-care-for-older-people-home-truths

p. 182 *'Complaints about home care to the ombudsman ...'* Ibid.

p. 182 *'delays in discharge have increased ...'* Nuffield Trust,
What are the Reasons for Delayed Transfers Of Care?,
29 October 2019, https://www.nuffieldtrust.org.uk/chart/
what-are-the-reasons-for-delayed-transfers-of-care

p. 187 *'an estimated annual revenue of nearly £16.9 billion ...'*
LaingBuisson, *Care Homes for Older People*, 24 July 2018, https://
www.laingbuisson.com/blog/laingbuisson-report-reappraises-
the-care-home-capacity-crisis-in-the-light-of-new-data/

p. 188 *'The* Financial Times *calculated in 2019 ...'* 'Britain's
Biggest Care Homes Rack up Debts of £40,000 a
Bed', *Financial Times*, July 2019, https://www.ft.com/
content/17c353c8-91b9-11e9-aea1-2b1d33ac3271

p. 188 *'a third of the UK's bed capacity ...'* *Care Markets*, December
2017/January 2018, https://www.laingbuisson.com/wpcontent/
uploads/2017/12/CareMarkets_Dec17Jan18.pdf

p. 188 *'Hull, for example, lost a third of its beds ...'* Incisive Health,
*Care Deserts: The Impact of a Dysfunctional Market in Adult Social
Care Provision*, May 2019, https://www.incisivehealth.com/wp-
content/uploads/2019/05/care-deserts-age-uk-report.pdf

p. 188 *'in poorer parts of the country ...'* Amelia Hill, 'UK Running
Out of Care Home Places', *Guardian*, 6 June 2019, https://www.
theguardian.com/society/2019/jun/06/uk-running-out-of-care-
home-places-says-geriatrics-society-chief

p. 189 *'In the 2019 election both Labour and Conservatives ...'* Labour
promised to double the number of people receiving free social
care, while the Conservatives pledged only to solve the social-
care crisis through cross-party consensus.

p. 189–90 *'England remains one of the few major advanced countries ...'*
Humphries, *Social Care*

p. 190   '*Scandinavian countries spend more than twice as much ...*'
          Bent Greve (ed.),'Long-term Care for the Elderly in Eleven
          European Countries', cited in ibid.

p. 190   '*Helping an elderly person to eat and swallow ...*' *The
          Cavendish Review*, July 2013, https://assets.publishing.service.
          gov.uk/government/uploads/system/uploads/attachment_data/
          file/236212/Cavendish_Review.pdf

p. 191   '*it will inflate local-authority costs ...*' Humphries, *Social
          Care*; also *Financial Times*, April 2017, https://www.ft.com/
          content/3eac5a0e-1536-11e7-80f4-13e067d5072c

p. 191   '*Glasgow council is due to pay £500 million ...*' 'Glasgow
          Council Carers "Could Quit" After Equal Pay Settlement',
          BBC News, 21 March 2019, https://www.bbc.co.uk/news/
          uk-scotland-glasgow-west-47652900

p. 191–2 '*2 per cent of directors of social services ...*' Humphries, *Social Care*

p. 192   '*the proportion paying for their care ...*' According to the King's
          Fund, exact figures on this are hard to work out, because there
          is no reliable data on total private expenditure on care.

p. 192   '*Research in the US ...*' US Department of Health and Human
          Services, *How Much Care Will You Need?*, https://longtermcare.
          acl.gov/the-basics/how-much-care-will-you-need.html

p. 197   '*There is no tradition of ageing wisely ...*' Chris Phillipson, *Ageing*
          (Polity Press, 2013)

p. 197   '*it is the fact that (with some exceptions) ...*' Royal Commission on
          Population, cited in ibid.

p. 198   '*enthusiasm, precision or a sense of priority ...*' Claire Hilton,
          Improving Psychiatric Care for Older People (Palgrave Macmillan,
          2017)

p. 198   '*the elderly bore their disappointment with dignity ...*' Charles
          Webster, *The NHS: A Political History*, Oxford University Press,
          2002

p. 198   *By the end of the 1950s ...*' Nicholas Timmins, *The Five Giants:
          A Biography of the Welfare State* (HarperCollins, 1995)

p. 198   '*It is not just the appearance ...*' Ibid.

p. 199   '*subdued and shaken by the stench ...*' Ibid.

p. 199   '*Another visitor to Friern Barnet ...*' Barbara Robb, *Sans
          Everything: A Case to Answer* (Nelson, 1967)

p. 199   *'Crossman admitted in his diaries ...'* Richard Crossman, *The Diaries of a Cabinet Minister*, Vol. 3 (Hamish Hamilton and Jonathan Cape, 1977)

p. 200   *'For one woman to suddenly do so much ...'* Brian Abel-Smith, interviewed by Hugh Freeman, *BJPsych Bulletin*, 1990.

p. 200   *'psychological experiments have shown ...'* John Kennedy, *John Kennedy's Care Home Inquiry*, Joseph Rowntree Foundation, 26 October 2014, https://www.jrf.org.uk/report/john-kennedys-care-home-inquiry

p. 205   *'Anguish has its own time-scale...'* John Berger, *A Fortunate Man: The Story of a Country Doctor* (Canongate, 2015)

(vi) dependence

p. 210   *'our own dependency...'* Eve Feder Kittay, *Love's Labor: Essays on Women, Equality and Dependency* (Routledge, 1999)

p. 210   *'Dependency is "a dirty word" in our society ...'* Jonathan Tomlinson, *A Better NHS*, https://abetternhs.net/about/

p. 211   *'life is lived from dependence to dependence...'* Henri Nouwen, *Our Greatest Gift: A Meditation on Caring and Dying* (HarperCollins, 1994)

p. 211   *'I shall look back on these days ...'* Cited in Royden R. Harrison, *The Life and Times of Sidney and Beatrice Webb, 1858–1905* (Palgrave Macmillan, 2000)

p. 211   *'she was a rare woman of her day ...'* Chris Renwick, *Bread for All: The Origins of the Welfare State* (Penguin, 2017)

7. The Ferryman's Task

p. 215   *'extended anthropological field trip...'* Robert Murphy, *The Body Silent: The Different World of the Disabled* (Henry Holt & Co., 1987)

p. 215   *'we are all born with two passports ...'* Susan Sontag, *Regarding the Pain of Others*, (Penguin, 2004)

p. 215   *'One's guides in this world have a dual role ...'* Cited in Seamus O'Mahony, *The Way We Die Now* (Head of Zeus, 2016)

p. 219   *'the stench of incontinence ...'* Julia Lawton, *The Dying Process* (Routledge, 2000)

p. 220   *'the only way to take the weight of my own mortality …'* Kevin Toolis, *My Father's Wake: How the Irish Teach Us to Live, Love and Die* (Weidenfeld & Nicolson, 2018)

p. 223   *'Philip Roth looked after his father …'* Philip Roth, *Patrimony: A True Story* (Simon and Schuster, 1991)

p. 227   *'Despite the popularity of hospices …'* Hospice UK, *Hospice Care in the UK 2016*, https://www.hospiceuk.org/docs/default-source/ What-We-Offer/publications-documents-and-files/hospice-care-in-the-uk-2016.pdf?sfvrsn=0

p. 227   *'over half of complaints to the NHS …'* 'Care of Dying Patients and Safety Dominate Complaints', *BMJ*, 10 February 2007, https://www.ncbi.nlm.nih.gov/pmc/articles/PMC1796720/

p. 228   *'Half a million people die every year …'* Office of National Statistics, https://www.ons.gov.uk/peoplepopulationandcommunity/ birthsdeathsandmarriages/deaths

p. 228   *'an extended period of frailty and vulnerability, lasting six years on average …'* Interview with Dr Caroline Nicholson, consultant in palliative care.

p. 229   *'A terminal prognosis should never include dates …'* Dr Karen Groves, Conference on Palliative Care, Crewe, 2017

p. 237   *'Parts of me died early on in my life …'* Jon Mooallem, 'One Man's Quest to Change the Way We Die', *New York Times*, 3 January 2017, https://www.nytimes.com/2017/01/03/magazine/ one-mans-quest-to-change-the-way-we-die.html

p. 237   *'There is a playfulness to perspective …'* Ibid.

p. 244   *'The Kerala Neighbourhood Network in Palliative Care …'* Suresh Kumar, 'Public Health Approaches to Palliative Care', *International Perspectives on Public Health and Palliative Care*, Libby Sallnow, et al. (eds.) (Routledge, 2012)

(vii) suffering

p. 247   *'Modern medical bureaucracy …'* Arthur Kleinman, *Illness Narratives: Suffering, Healing and the Human Condition* (Basic Books, 1988)

p. 247   *'Pain is a sensation …'* Cited in James Davies, *The Importance of Suffering: The Value and Meaning of Emotional Discontent* (Routledge, 2011)

p. 248   '*the underworld of suffering . . .*' Henry Marsh, *Admissions: A Life in Brain Surgery* (Weidenfeld & Nicolson, 2017)

p. 248   '*empathic witnessing . . .*' Kleinman, *Illness Narratives*

p. 249   '*both sets and reflects standards . . .*' Arthur Frank, *The Renewal of Generosity: Illness, Medicine and How to Live* (University of Chicago Press, 2004)

8. Possible Futures

p. 254   '*rising productivity would increase wealth threefold . . .*' Cited in Julian Tudor Hart, *The Political Economy of Healthcare* (Policy Press, 2010)

p. 254   '*From its inception, the NHS attracted . . .*' Patrick Butler, 'How migrants helped make the NHS', *Guardian*, 18 June 2008, https://www.theguardian.com/society/2008/jun/18/nhs60.nhs2

p. 255   '*In 2012 over a fifth of the UK's nurses . . .*' ONS, *International Migration and the Healthcare Workforce*, 15 August 2019, https://www.ons.gov.uk/peoplepopulationandcommunity/populationandmigration/internationalmigration/articles/internationalmigrationandthehealthcareworkforce/2019-08-15

p. 255   '*13.1 per cent of all NHS . . .*' Carl Baker, *One NHS: Many Nationalities: 2017*, House of Commons Library, 19 October 2017, https://commonslibrary.parliament.uk/social-policy/health/one-nhs-many-nationalities-2017/

p. 255   '*The comparable figures in France or Italy are much smaller . . .*' OECD, 'Foreign-trained Doctors and Nurses', *Health at a Glance 2017*, https://www.oecd-ilibrary.org/docserver/health_glance-2017-59-en.pdf?expires=1580487457&id=id&accname=guest&checksum=F8C2A3BFFBB6DB1FA6420DA775A575E1

p. 255   '*one fifth of all UK care workers were born abroad . . .*' Independent Age, *Moved to Care: The Impact of Migration on the Adult Social Care Workforce*, https://independent-age-assets.s3.eu-west-1.amazonaws.com/s3fs-public/2016-05/IA%20Moved%20to%20care%20report_12%2011%2015.pdf

p. 255   '*more than half of all care workers . . .*' Ibid.

p. 255   '*a significant number of EU nationals have left . . .*' Michael Savage, 'NHS Winter Crisis Fears Grow After Thousands of

EU Staff Quit', *Guardian*, 24 November 2019, citing Liberal Democrat research that 11,600 EU NHS staff have left since the Brexit vote in 2016, https://www.theguardian.com/society/2019/nov/24/nhs-winter-crisis-thousands-eu-staff-quit; also figures from the Nursing and Midwifery Council show that the number of nurses arriving from the EU dropped by 87 per cent from 6,382 in 2016–17 to 805 in 2017–18, https://www.nmc.org.uk/news/news-and-updates/new-nmc-figures-continue-to-highlight-major-concern-as-more-eu-nurses-leave-the-uk/

p. 256   '*robots are increasingly used in surgery* ...' Taxpayers' Alliance, *Automate the State: Better and Cheaper Public Services*, 20 June 2019, https://www.taxpayersalliance.com/automate_the_state_better_and_cheaper_public_services

p. 256   '*Google DeepMind has started using AI* ...' Ibid.; also 'Using AI to Plan Head and Neck Cancer Treatments', *DeepMind*, September 2018, https://deepmind.com/blog/article/ai-uclh-radiotherapy-planning

p. 256   '*a Danish software company applied* ...' 'AI That Detects Cardiac Arrests During Emergency Calls Will Be Tested Across Europe This Summer', *The Verge*, April 2018, https://www.theverge.com/2018/4/25/17278994/ai-cardiac-arrest-corti-emergency-call-response

p. 257   '*Advances in the technology* ...' UK-RAS Network, *Robotics in Social Care: A Connected Care Ecosystem for Independent Living*, 2017, https://www.ukras.org/wp-content/uploads/2018/10/UK_RAS_wp_social_spread_low_res_ref.pdf

p. 258   '*Around £3.6 billion has already been invested* ...' Malcolm Foster, 'Aging Japan: Robots May Have Role in Future of Elder Care', *Reuters*, 27 March 2018, https://www.reuters.com/article/us-japan-ageing-robots-widerimage/aging-japan-robots-may-have-role-in-future-of-elder-care-idUSKBN1H33AB

p. 258   '*One robot developed for the Japanese market* ...' Riken press release, 2015, https://www.riken.jp/en/news_pubs/research_news/2015/20150223_2/

p. 258   '*one influential report* ...' Ara Darzi, et al., *Better Health and Care for All: A Ten-Point Plan for the 2020s*, IPPR,

15 June 2018, https://www.ippr.org/research/publications/better-health-and-care-for-all

p. 260   '*This is not about either technology or relationship* . . .' Valerie Iles, 'Why Reforming The NHS Doesn't Work: The Importance of Understanding How Good People Offer Bad Care', *Really Learning*, 2011

p. 260   '*Another enthusiastic report* . . .' Taxpayers' Alliance, *Automate the State*

p. 261   '*we consider it essential that* . . .' UK-RAS Network, *Robotics in Social Care*

p. 261   '*a flight from conversation* . . .' Sherry Turkle, *Alone Together* (Basic Books, 2011)

p. 261   '*In a groundbreaking study of nurses* . . .' Isabel Menzies Lyth, *Social Systems as a Defense Against Anxiety*, 1960, http://www.moderntimesworkplace.com/archives/ericsess/sessvol1/Lythp439.opd.pdf

p. 262   '*disturbing tension that can be aroused* . . .' Adam Phillips and Barbara Taylor, *On Kindness* (Hamish Hamilton, 2009)

p. 262   '*Turkle likens the impact of technology* . . .' Sherry Turkle, *Reclaiming Conversation: The Power of Talk in a Digital Age* (Penguin, 2015)

p. 263   '*the human brain has two contrasting ways* . . .' Iain McGilchrist, *The Master and His Emissary: The Divided Brain and the Making of the Western World* (Yale University Press, 2015)

p. 263   '*more accurate, more down to earth* . . .' Iain McGilchrist in conversation with Jonathan Rowson, *Divided Brain, Divided World*, RSA, 1 February 2013, https://www.thersa.org/discover/publications-and-articles/reports/divided-brain-divided-world

p. 264   '*A famous psychological experiment* . . .' Daniel Simons and Christopher Chabris, *Selective Attention Test*, 1999, https://www.youtube.com/watch?v=vJG698U2Mvo

p. 264   '*the nature of the attention we choose* . . .' McGilchrist and Rowson, *Divided Brain*

p. 265   '*we expect more from technology* . . .' Sherry Turkle, 'The Flight from Conversation', *New York Times*, 21 April 2012, https://www.nytimes.com/2012/04/22/opinion/sunday/the-flight-from-conversation.html

p. 265   *'There are estimated to be 150,000 therapists ...'* Figure used by
            BBC, 2009; see also Debbie Sharp, et al., 'Complementary
            Medicine Use, Views and Experiences: A National Survey in
            England', *BJGP Open*, 2:4, December 2018, https://www.ncbi.
            nlm.nih.gov/pmc/articles/PMC6348322/

p. 265   *'automation will be rapid ...'* Adair Turner, *Capitalism in the Age
            of Robots: Work, Income and Wealth in the 21st Century*, lecture at
            Johns Hopkins University, Washington DC, 10 April 2018

p. 266   *'There has been a 20 per cent growth ...'* Shereen Hussein,
            PSSRU, January 2019, https://www.pssru.ac.uk/our-people/
            shereen-hussein/?page=all

p. 266   *'there will be a profound shift ...'* Andy Haldane, *Ideas and
            Institutions: A Growth Story*, speech at Oxford University,
            2018, https://www.bankofengland.co.uk/-/media/boe/files/
            speech/2018/ideas-and-institutions-a-growth-story-speech-
            by-andy-haldane

p. 267   *'caring will be one of the great professions ...'* Martin
            Rees, 'How Soon Will Robots Overtake the World?',
            Daily Telegraph, 23 May 2015, https://www.telegraph.co.uk/
            culture/hay-festival/11605785/Astronomer-Royal-Martin-Rees-
            predicts-the-world-will-be-run-by-computers-soon.html

p. 270   *'If you want to be a pedagogue you ...'* Cited in Gabriel Eichsteller
            and Sylvia Holthoff, *The Art of Being a Social Pedagogue: Practice
            Examples of Cultural Change in Children's Homes in Essex*,
            Essex County Council, http://www.thempra.org.uk/downloads/
            Essex_Report_2012.pdf

p. 271   *'Social pedagogy recognizes the need for spontaneity ...'* Ibid.

p. 271   *'Schwartz Rounds ...'* Point of Care Foundation, https://www.
            pointofcarefoundation.org.uk/our-work/schwartz-rounds/

p. 271   *'Shared Lives Plus ...'* Shared Lives Plus, https://sharedlives-
            plus.org.uk

p. 272   *'Social prescribing is a scheme ...'* King's Fund, *What is Social
            Prescribing?*, 2 February 2017, https://www.kingsfund.org.uk/
            publications/social-prescribing

p. 272   *'Other countries have experimented ...'* David Halpern, *The
            Hidden Wealth of Humans* (Polity Press, 2010)

p. 273   *'the Women's Budget Group calculated ...'* De Henau, et al., *Investing in the Care Economy*, 2016, https://wbg.org. uk/wp-content/uploads/2016/11/De_Henau_Perrons_WBG_ CareEconomy_ITUC_briefing_final.pdf

p. 273 *'foundational economy ...'* Justin Bentham, et al., *Manifesto for the Foundational Economy*, CRESC Working Paper 131, November 2013, http://hummedia.manchester.ac.uk/institutes/ cresc/workingpapers/wp131.pdf

p. 274 *'The ideas have been taken up by the Welsh government ...'* Lee Waters, *Foundational Economy*, 15 February 2019, https://gov. wales/written-statement-foundational-economy

p. 274 *'we need to start from an argument ...'* Bentham, et al., *Manifesto for the Foundational Economy*

p. 275 *'such systems of meaning may fragment ...'* Yuval Harari, *Homo Deus* (HarperCollins, 2017)

p. 276 *'the dilemmas of the artist ...'* Lewis Hyde, *The Gift* (Penguin, 2007)

p. 277 *'a fundamental truth of human existence ...'* Richard Titmuss, *The Gift Relationship: From Human Blood to Social Policy* (Allen and Unwin, 1970)

p. 278 *'The gift economy of many indigenous ...'* Marcel Mauss, *The Gift* (1925; English translation, W.W. Norton & Co., 1954)

Select Bibliography

Avent, Ryan, *The Wealth of Humans, Work and its Absence in the Twenty First Century*, 2016, Allen Lane

Ballat, John, and Campling, Penelope, *Intelligent Kindness: Reforming the Culture of Healthcare*, 2011, RCPsych Publications

Baraitser, Lisa, *Maternal Encounters: The Ethics of Interruption*, 2008, Routledge

Benn, Melissa, *What Should We Tell Our Daughters? The Pleasures and Pressures of Growing up Female*, 2013, Hodder & Stoughton

Benn, Melissa, *Madonna and Child: The Politics of Modern Motherhood*, 1998, Jonathan Cape

Bennett, Alan, *The Lady in the Van*, 1999, Profile Books

Berger, John, *A Fortunate Man: The Story of a Country Doctor*, 2015, Canongate

Borsay, Anne, *Disability and Social Policy in Britain since 1750*, 2004, Palgrave

Bostridge, Mark, *Florence Nightingale*, 2008, Viking

Brown, Guy, *The Living End: The Future of Death, Aging and Immortality*, 2007, Macmillan Science

Brykczynska, Gosia, *Caring: The Compassion and Wisdom of Nursing*, 1996, CRC Press

Bryson, Valerie, *Gender and the Politics of Time*, 2007, Policy Press

Burggraf, Shirley P., *The Feminine Economy and Economic Man: Reviving the Role of Family in the Post Industrial Age*, 1995, Basic Books

Carr, Nicholas, *The Shallows*, 2011, W. W. Norton & Co.

Case, Molly, *How to Treat People: A Nurse at Work*, 2019, Viking

Casell, E. J., *The Nature of Suffering and the Goals of Medicine*, 2004, Oxford University Press

Cottam, Hilary, *Radical Help*, 2018, Virago

Coutts, Marion, *The Iceberg: A Memoir*, 2014, Atlantic

Dalley, Gillian, *Ideologies of Caring: Rethinking Community and Collectivism*, 1996, Palgrave

Daly, Mary, and Rake, Katherine, *Gender and the Welfare State: Care Work and Welfare in Europe and the USA*, 2003, Polity Press

Davies, James, *The Importance of Suffering: The Value and Meaning of Emotional Discontent*, 2011, Routledge

De Beauvoir, Simone, *The Second Sex*, 2015, Vintage

Feder Kittay, Eve, *Love's Labor: Essays on Women, Equality and Dependency*, 1999, Routledge

Folbre, Nancy, *The Invisible Heart: Economics and Family Values*, 2001, New Press

Ford, Martin, *The Rise of the Robots, Technology and the Threat of Mass Unemployment*, 2015, Oneworld

Finch, Janet, and Groves, Dulcie (eds) *A Labour of Love: Women, Work and Caring*, 1983, Routledge & Kegan Paul

Frank, Arthur, *The Renewal of Generosity: Illness, Medicine and How to Live*, 2004, University of Chicago Press

Fraser, Nancy, *Fortunes of Feminism: From Women's Liberation to Identity Politics to Anti-capitalism*, 2013, Verso

Freely, Maureen, *What About Us? An Open Letter to the Mothers Feminism Forgot*, 1995, Bloomsbury

Friedan, Betty, *The Feminine Mystique*, 2015, Penguin

Gawande, Atul, *Being Mortal: Illness, Medicine and What Matters in the End*, 2015, Profile Books

Gerrard Nicci, *What Dementia Teaches Us About Love*, 2019, Allen Lane

Gilligan, Carol, *In a Different Voice: Psychological Theory and Women's Development*, 1990, Harvard University Press

Gordon, Suzanne, *Nursing Against the Odds*, 2006, Cornell

Halpern, David, *The Hidden Wealth of Humans*, 2010, Polity Press

Hamington, Maurice, *Embodied Care*, 2004, University of Illinois Press

Harari, Yuval, *Homo Deus*, 2017, HarperCollins USA

Harrison, R., *The Life and Times of Sidney and Beatrice Webb*, 2000, Palgrave Macmillan

Himmelweit, S. (ed.), *Inside the Household: From Labour to Care*, 2016, Palgrave Macmillan

Himmelweit, S., and Plomien, A., 'Feminist Perspectives on Care', in Mary Evans, et al. (ed.) *The Sage Handbook of Feminist Theory*, 2014, Sage

Hays, Sharon, *The Cultural Contradictions of Motherhood*, 1998, Yale University Press

Heath, Iona: *The Mystery of General Practice*, 1995, Nuffield Trust, https://www.nuffieldtrust.org.uk/research/the-mystery-of-general-practice

Held, Virginia, *The Ethics of Care: Personal, Political and Global*, 2005, Oxford University Press

Hilton, Claire, *Improving Psychiatric Care for Older People*, 2017, Palgrave Macmillan

Hochschild, Arlie Russell, *The Commercialization of Intimate Life*, 2003, University of California Press

Hollway, Wendy, *The Capacity to Care*, 2006, Routledge

Howarth, Glennys, *Death and Dying: A Sociological Introduction*, 2006, Polity Press

Hyde, Lewis, *The Gift*, 2007, Penguin Random House, USA

Ignatieff, Michael, *The Needs of Strangers*, 1985, Viking

Iliffe, Steve, *From General Practice to Primary Care: The Industrialization of Family Medicine*, 2008, Oxford University Press, USA

Ismay, Penelope, *Trust Among Strangers, Friendly Societies in Modern Britain*, 2018, Cambridge University Press

Karpf, Anne, *How to Age* (The School of Life), 2014, Macmillan

Kellehear, Allan, *A Social History of Dying*, 2007, Cambridge University Press

Kellehear, Allan, *Compassionate Cities: Public Health and End-of-life Care*, 2005, Routledge

Kleinman, Arthur, *Illness Narratives: Suffering, Healing and the Human Condition*, 1988, Basic Books

Lawton, Julia, *The Dying Process*, 2000, Routledge

Leadbeater, Charles, and Garber, Jake, *Dying for a Change*, 2010, Demos

Lethbridge, Lucy, *Servants: A Downstairs View of Twentieth-century Britain*, 2013, Bloomsbury

Marçal, Katrine, *Who Cooked Adam Smith's Dinner?*, 2015, Granta

Marquand, David, *Mammon Kingdom: An Essay on Britain, Now*, 2014, Allen Lane

Marsh, Henry, *Admissions: A Life in Brain Surgery*, 2017, Weidenfeld & Nicolson

McGilchrist, Iain, *The Master and His Emissary: The Divided Brain and the Making of the Western World*, 2015, Yale University Press

McKenna, Hugh, *Nursing Theories and Models*, 1997, Routledge

McRobbie, Angela, *The Aftermath of Feminism: Gender, Culture and Social Change*, 2008, Sage

Mol, Annemarie, *The Logic of Care: Health and the Problem of Patient Choice*, 2008, Routledge

Morris Jnr, Roy, *The Better Angel: Walt Whitman in the Civil War*, 2000, Oxford University Press, USA

Murphy, Robert, *The Body Silent: The Different World of the Disabled*, 1987, Henry Holt & Co.

Nelson Siobhan, *Say Little, Do Much: Nursing, Nuns and Hospital in the Nineteenth Century*, 2001, University of Pennsylvania Press

Nelson, Siobhan, and Gordon, Suzanne (eds) *The Complexities of Care: Nursing Reconsidered*, 2000, Cornell

Noddings, Nel, *Caring: A Feminine Approach to Ethics and Moral Education*, 2013, University of California Press

Nouwen, Henri, *Our Greatest Gift: A Meditation on Caring and Dying*, 1994, HarperCollins

Nussbaum, Martha, *Political Emotions: Why Love Matters for Justice*, 2013, Belknap Press

O'Mahony, Seamus, *The Way We Die Now*, 2016, Head of Zeus

Patel, Raj, and Moore, Jason W., *A History of the World in Seven Cheap Things*, 2018, Verso

Phillips, Adam, and Taylor, Barbara, *On Kindness*, 2009, Hamish Hamilton

Phillips, Judith, *Care*, 2007, Polity Press

Phillipson, Chris, *Ageing*, 2013, Polity Press

Pierson, John, *Understanding Social Work: History and Context*, 2011, Open University Press

Prochaska, Frank, *Christianity and Social Services in Britain: The Disinherited Spirit*, 2008, Oxford University Press

Rafferty, Anne Marie, et al., *An Introduction to the Social History of Nursing*, 1988, Routledge

Rafferty, Anne Marie, *The Politics of Nursing Knowledge*, 1996, Routledge

Raverat Darwin, Gwen, *Period Piece: A Cambridge Childhood*, 1952, Faber

Renwick, Chris, *Bread for All: The Origins of the Welfare State*, 2017, Penguin

Rich, Adrienne, *On Lies, Secrets and Silence*, 1979, W. W. Norton & Co.

Ruddick, Sara, *Maternal Thinking: Towards a Politics of Peace*, 1995, Beacon Press

Robb, Barbara, *Sans Everything: A Case to Answer*, 1967, Nelson

Roth, Philip, *Patrimony: A True Story*, 1991, Simon and Schuster

Runciman, David, *How Democracy Ends*, 2018, Profile

Sandel, Michael, *What Money Can't Buy: The Moral Limits of Markets*, 2012, Farrar Straus Giroux

Saunders, Cicely, *Selected Writings, 1958–2004*, 2006, Oxford University Press

Sevenhuijsen, Selma, *Citizenship and the Ethics of Care*, 1998, Routledge

Smith, Pam, *The Emotional Cost of Nursing Revisited: Can Nurses Still Care?*, 2011, Palgrave

Sontag, Susan, *Regarding the Pain of Others*, 2004, Penguin (new edn)

Tallis, Raymond, *Hippocratic Oaths: Medicine and Its Discontents*, 2004, Atlantic

Thane, Pat, and Botelho, Lynn, *The Long History of Old Age*, 2005, Thames and Hudson

Thomson, Rachel, *Making Modern Mothers*, 2011, Policy Press

Timmins Nicholas, *Five Giants: A Biography of the Welfare State*, 1995, HarperCollins

Titmuss, Richard, *The Gift Relationship: From Human Blood to Social Policy*, 1970, Allen and Unwin

Tolstoy, Leo, *The Death of Ivan Ilyich*, 1886; 2008, Penguin

Tomlinson, John, *The Culture of Speed: The Coming of Immediacy*, 2007, Sage

Toolis, Kevin, *My Father's Wake: How the Irish Teach Us to Live, Love and Die*, 2018, Weidenfeld & Nicolson

Tronto, Joan, *Moral Boundaries: A Political Argument for an Ethic of Care*, 1993, Routledge

Tudor Hart, Julian, *The Political Economy of Health Care*, 2010, Policy Press

Turkle, Sherry, *Alone Together*, 2011, Basic Books

Watson, Christie, *The Language of Kindness: A Nurse's Story*, 2018, Chatto & Windus

Wolf, Alison, *XX Factor: How Working Women are Creating a New Society*, 2013, Profile

Woolf, Virginia, *On Being Ill*, 1930, Hogarth Press; 2002, Paris Press

Woolf, Virginia, 'Professions for Women', in *The Death of the Moth and Other Essays*, 1942; http://gutenberg.net.au/ebooks12/1203811h.html

Index